KETO CHAFFLE COOKBOOK

100 EASY AND TASTY LOW-CARB RECIPES TO HELP YOU LIVE HEALTHILY AND LOSE WEIGHT WHILE HAVING FUN MAKING DELICIOUS KETO WAFFLES

BY SUSAN LOMBARDI

Disclaimer

All erudition supplied in this book is specified for educational and academic purpose only. The author is not in any way in charge for any outcomes that emerge from utilizing this book. Constructive efforts have been made to render information that is both precise and effective, however the author is not to be held answerable for the accuracy or use/misuse of this information.

TABLE OF CONTENTS

INTRODUCTION

In the low carb/keto setting, chaffles have become an instant phenomenon. The addition of almond flour transforms them into more conventional waffles, which are almost entirely made of cheese and eggs. Their amusing name combines the words "cheese" and "waffle." Last year, chaffles became popular as a low-carb, keto-friendly treat. In reality, chaffle recipes were one of the most sought-after recipes in 2019!

So there are a few different chaffle recipes floating about, but the basic recipe calls for an egg and cheddar cheese. To make a chaffle from the original recipes, no baking soda is needed.

CHAPTER ONE

WHAT IS A CHAFFLE?

A chaffle's basic ingredients are cheddar cheese, almond flour, and an egg. In a mixing bowl, combine all of the ingredients and pour on top of your waffle maker. After this chaffle recipe went viral the other day, waffle makers are possibly on the rise right now. I was cynical at first, thinking there was no way this could work after mixing it together and pouring the batter over the waffle. I was anticipating massive shambles. Make sure the waffle maker is well sprayed. The waffle turned out beautifully, with a crispy exterior and a fluffy inside.

THERE ARE TWO INGREDIENTS IN THIS CHAFFLE RECIPE.

One of the reasons I was interested in trying this chaffle recipe was that it only needed two ingredients: cheese and eggs. There are, however, other recipes that include sweeteners, almond flour, and other ingredients.

WHAT IS A CHAFFLE AND HOW DO I MAKE ONE?

A good waffle iron is needed to make a chaffle. This is one of my favorites. The Villaware Belgian waffle maker is what it's called. I'm a big fan of Alton Brown's show, and I have the same waffle iron he does.

If your waffle maker needs it, preheat it.

In a mixing bowl, whisk together the milk, cheddar, and almond flour until well mixed.

After spraying the waffle maker with cooking spray, add the chaffle batter on top. Close the waffle maker and set it aside for 3 to 4 minutes. My waffle maker has its own built-in automatic timer.

Remove the waffle from the waffle iron and serve.

WHAT WOULD A CHAFFLE BE USED FOR?

I saw this served with sausage gravy on the keto recipes subreddit, and it looked like pure heaven. You may use the recipe to make burger buns, pizza crust, breakfast sandwiches, and so on. This recipe can be used for a variety of purposes, and i plan to make more.

CAN CHAFFLES BE FREEZED?

They do freeze well. To keep them fresh for longer, wrap them tightly in plastic wrap and store them in an airtight container. They can be frozen for up to a month. I haven't done any more testing than that.

IS IT POSSIBLE TO PRODUCE CHAFFLES THROUGHOUT THE WHOLE WEEK AT ONCE?

You can also make fresh chaffles for the week by preparing ahead of time. As long as you keep them refrigerated, they can remain fresh. To reheat them, simply heat them in the microwave or an air fryer. If you're looking for a crispy result, the air fryer is the way to go!

CHAFFLE SUGGESTIONS

Keep in mind that this is only a starting point. You may omit any ingredient or substitute different types of cheese. Mozzarella also works. Use a dairy-free cheese like Daiya if you have a dairy allergy.

One chaffle is made from the whole recipe.

Allow chaffles to cool fully before putting them in the freezer. It's easy to prepare ahead of time for meal prep. To keep them fresh during the week, store them in airtight containers.

CHAPTER TWO

WHAT'S THE KETO DIET?

The keto diet is highly low in carbs, which can be difficult to stick to in general, but particularly when cravings for diner-style pancakes and french toast arise. Two slices of french toast have about 30 grams of net carbs, which is more than many keto dieters can consume in a single day. That's not going to work, unfortunately.

The cheese waffle, also known as a "chaffle," is a keto-friendly waffle made with eggs and cheese. They're a filling option that's also easy to produce, which isn't true of all keto recipe swaps. (see also: keto diet breakfast ideas that will make you jump out of bed)

To make chaffles, you won't need an inventory of specialty keto ingredients. A chaffle is simply a mixture of eggs and mozzarella cheese at its most simple level. Mozzarella is a relatively benign cheese (in the sense that it does not have the pungent taste that other cheeses do). It also melts well, which is important in this recipe. Almond flour is used in this chaffles recipe to give it a more typical waffle-like feel. Since it's high in fat and low in net carbs, it's an ingredient you'll want to stock up on if you're on a keto diet. (see also: vegan keto recipes that show there's more to keto than bacon)

WHAT IS THE KETO DIET, EXACTLY?

According to Scott Keatley, RD, of Keatley Medical Nutrition Therapy, this eating plan is all about limiting carbs and increasing fats to get the body to use fat as a source of energy.

Although each person's body and needs are unique, this usually translates to:

- Fat accounts for 60 to 75 percent of your calories, while protein accounts for 15 to 30 percent.
- Carbohydrates should account for 5 to 10% of your total calories.
- This typically entails consuming no more than 50 grams of carbohydrates a day (some strict keto dieters even opt for just 20 grams a day).

HOW DID THE KETOGENIC DIET COME TO BE?

According to New York-based RD Jessica Cording, the keto diet was initially created to support people with seizure disorders, not to help people lose weight. This is because ketones and another chemical released by the diet, beta-hydroxybutyrate, can both help to reduce seizure frequency.

KETO DIET WITH A CYCLIC PATTERN

"The cyclic keto diet is similar to normal keto, only one to two days a week," Rissetto says. "A cyclic keto dieter can follow traditional keto recommendations five to six days per week. They would then have a 'carb loop,' also known as a 'carb refeed,' for one or two days. They will consume approximately 140 to 160 grams of carbohydrates on this day. "

Athletes also adopt this form of keto diet because they need a carb to refeed day to replenish glycogen reserves in their muscles. "High-intensity physical exercise depletes almost all of the glycogen stored in their muscles, necessitating replenishment," says Rissetto.

It's worth remembering, though, that just because you want to follow this diet doesn't mean you have to eat a lot of processed foods and desserts on your days off. Instead, get your carbs from whole grains, starchy vegetables, and fruits.

KETO DIET WITH A SPECIFIC GOAL

"On this diet, you meet all of the rules of the traditional keto diet, with one exception: you consume carbohydrates before intense workouts," Rissetto states. "About 30 minutes to an hour before working out, targeted keto dieters will eat anything from 25 to 50 grams of carbohydrates. Dieters also report feeling better and more capable during workouts as a result of this.

Although this will momentarily knock you out of ketosis, it will return within a few hours, depending on how many carbs you ate." The reasoning behind this diet is that since the extra carbs are burned off right away, they won't be retained as body fat.

Here it comes with a variety of keto chaffle recipes in the next Chapter.

BREAKFAST RECIPES

CHAFFLES

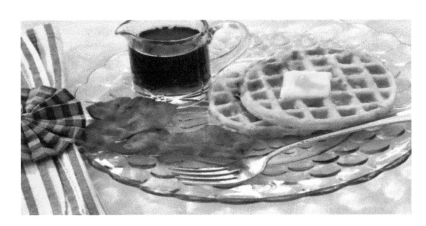

Time required: 20 min

Portions provided: 2

Ingredients:

- 1 large egg

- ½ cup shredded mozzarella cheese

Preparation:

1. Waffle iron should be preheated.

2. Whisk together the egg and mozzarella cheese in a small cup.

3. Pour half of the batter into the waffle maker and spread it out from the middle with a spoon. Close the waffle maker and cook for 3 minutes, or until the steaming has stopped and the chaffle has browned well. A chewy texture may result from overcooking. Repeat the procedure with the remaining batter.

Nutrition Facts: *Per Serving:* Calories 108; Protein 10g; Carbohydrates 1g; Fat 7g; Cholesterol 111.1mg; Sodium 209.9mg.

PUMPKIN CHAFFLES

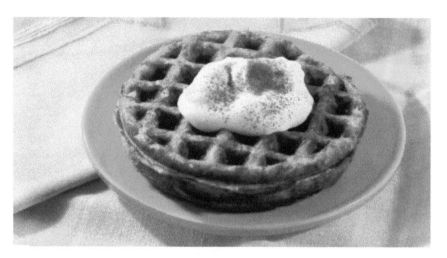

Time required: 20 min

Portions provided: 2

Ingredients:

- ¼ cup pumpkin puree
- 1 egg
- 1 teaspoon maple extract
- ½ cup shredded mozzarella cheese
- 1 tablespoon almond flour
- ¾ teaspoon pumpkin pie spice
- ¼ teaspoon baking powder
- Whipped Cream:
- ¼ cup heavy cream
- ½ teaspoon granulated erythritol sweetener (such as Swerve®)
- ¼ teaspoon maple extract
- 1 pinch ground cinnamon (Optional)

Preparation:

1. Pre - heat a waffle maker according to the manufacturer's instructions.
2. Combine the pumpkin puree, egg, and maple extract in a small mixing bowl. In a big mixing bowl, combine the mozzarella cheese, almond flour, pumpkin pie spice, and baking powder.
3. With a spoon, spread 1/2 of the batter out from the center of the preheated waffle maker (don't overfill or the waffle maker will overflow). Cook for 3 to 4 minutes, or until the steaming stops and the chaffle reaches your desired doneness. Repeat with the remaining batter after removing the waffle maker from the oven. Allow to cool slightly as you prepare the whipped cream.
4. Fill a small mixing bowl halfway with heavy cream and whisk for 1 to 2 minutes, or until soft peaks form. Decrease the frequency to low and add the sweetener, whisking constantly until stiff peaks form.
5. Place 1 chaffle on a plate, top with whipped cream, and a sprinkle of cinnamon to serve.

Nutrition Facts: *Per Serving:* Calories 255; Protein 11.8g; Carbohydrates 7.2g; Fat 20.1g; Cholesterol 151.8mg; Sodium 356.5mg.

BURGER BUN CHAFFLE

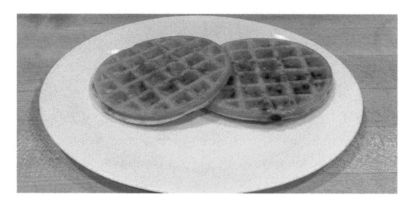

Time required: 5 min

Portions provided: 2

Ingredients:

- 1 large egg, beaten
- 1/2 cup shredded mozzarella
- 1 TB almond flour
- 1/4 tsp baking powder
- 1 tsp sesame seeds
- 1 Pinch of onion powder

Preparation:

1. Combine all ingredients in a mixing bowl.
2. Pour half of the batter into a mini waffle maker (or split between two)
3. Cook for 5 minutes, or until the waffle maker is no longer producing steam.
4. Enable to cool fully on a wire rack.

Nutrition Facts: Calories 137; Total Carbs 2g; Net Carbs 2g; Fat 12g; Protein 10g.

BACONY CARNIVORE WOMELETTES

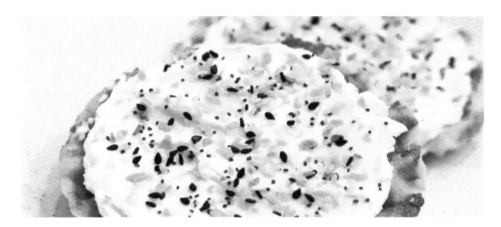

Time required: 10 min

Portions provided: 1

Ingredients:

- 1 slice bacon, raw
- 1 egg, large
- splash maple extract, if desired
- hefty pinch of any spices or flavorings you'd like, as desired

Preparation:

1. Switch on the blender or food processor with the bacon.
2. Put the egg and any seasonings down the chute until the bacon is mostly ground up and continue to operate the machine until liquified and well-incorporated. This is your slurry of womelette.
3. Heat your mini-waffle maker according to the manufacturer's instructions.
4. Half of the slurry should be poured into the waffle maker, and the lid should be closed.
5. Cook until golden brown or until cooked to your liking, around 3-5 minutes.
6. Remove the waffle maker from the oven and repeat steps 4 and 5 with the rest of the slurry.
7. Warmth can be enjoyed in a variety of ways.

Nutrition Facts: *Per a womelette*: Calories 59; Protein 4.4g; Fat 4.4g; Carbs 0.3g; Fiber 0g; Sugar 0g

KETO WAFFLES

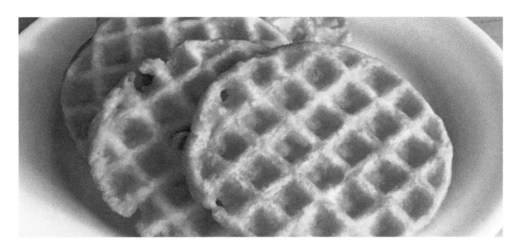

Time required: 30 min

Portions provided: 5

Ingredients:

- 5 eggs - medium separated
- 4 tbsp coconut flour
- 4 tbsp granulated sweetener of choice or more, to taste
- 1 tsp baking powder
- 2 tsp vanilla
- 3 tbsp full fat milk or cream
- 125 g (1 stick plus 1 tbsp) butter melted

Preparation:

1. This is the first cup.
2. Whisk the egg whites until they are rigid and firm.
3. Bowl No. 2
4. Combine the egg yolks, coconut flour, sweetener, and baking powder in a large mixing bowl.
5. Slowly drizzle in the melted butter, stirring constantly to maintain a smooth consistency.
6. Mix in the milk and vanilla extract thoroughly.
7. Fold spoonfuls of whisked egg whites into the yolk mixture gently. Attempt to retain as much air and fluffiness as possible.
8. Fill the warm waffle maker halfway with the waffle batter to make one waffle. Cook, stirring occasionally, until golden brown.
9. Rep until you've used up half of the mixture.

CHAFFLE KETO WITHOUT DAIRY

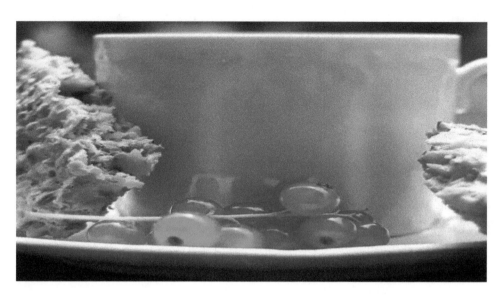

Time required: 3 min

Portions provided: 3

Ingredients:

- 1 tablespoon coconut flour
- 1 tablespoon beef gelatin powder
- A pinch of salt
- 2 large eggs
- 1 tablespoon of mayonnaise

Preparation:

1. In a small cup, combine the coconut flour, beef gelatine, and salt.
2. In a separate bowl, whisk together the eggs and mayonnaise. Avocado oil spray should be sprayed on the waffle iron.
3. Divide the batter into thirds and pour one-third of a serving into the waffle iron.
4. Wait about 2 minutes for the light to go out after closing the lid. Make sure it's perfect the way you like it. Place the waffle iron on a plate and re-spray it with cooking spray. Repeat with the remaining two batter servings.
5. Enjoy right now, or store in the fridge for later use in a sandwich.

Nutrition Facts: Net Carbohydrates: 1g; Calories 109 calories from fat 72; Fat 8g12%; Saturated fat 2g13%; Cholesterol 146mg 49%; 202mg Sodium 9%; Potassium 52mg 1%;

Carbohydrates 2g1%; Fiber 1g4%; Sugar 1g1%; Protein 7g14%; Calcium 21 mg2%; Iron 1 mg6% *

daily percentages are based on a 2,000 calorie diet.

PALEO COCONUT FLOUR PODS

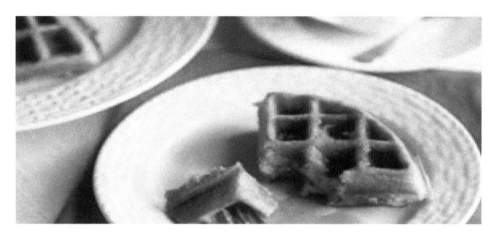

Time required: 7 min

Portions provided: 4

Ingredients:

- 4 tablespoons of melted butter or paleo ghee
- 6 eggs see note
- ⅛ teaspoon of optional stevia sweetleaf drops or 2 sachets of sweetener
- ½ teaspoon of salt
- ½ teaspoon of baking powder
- ⅓ cup of coconut flour 33 grams

Preparation:

1. In a blender, combine the butter and eggs until thoroughly combined.
2. Mix in the stevia, salt, and yeast.
3. Apply the coconut flour and stir until it is fully lump-free. Allow for at least five minutes of resting time for the dough to thicken.
4. To dilute the batter, add a little water as needed.
5. Waffles should be cooked according to the waffle iron's instructions.

Notes:

1. You may also use coconut oil instead of butter or clarified butter.

2. You may use cream, almond milk, or coconut milk instead of one or two eggs. 3–4 tablespoons of liquid are needed to replace an egg.

3. Where possible, weigh the coconut flour instead of using a cup calculation because the cup measurement isn't as precise. You can need to use a little less flour if the waffles are dry, and a little more if the batter is too thin, due to the absorbency of the flour. To smooth out a thick batter, you can add more liquid.

CHAFFLE WITHOUT EGG

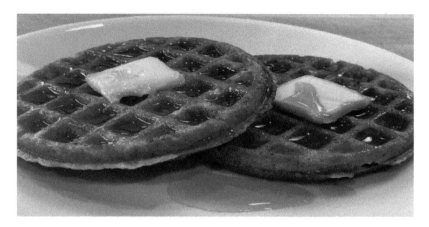

Time required: 10 min

Portions provided: 2

Ingredients:

- 2 tb of almond flour
- 1 tb of coconut flour
- 1 tb whey protein isolate (see notes)
- 1 teaspoon "pixie dust" (see notes)
- 1/4 teaspoon of xanthan gum
- 1/4 cup mozzarella, mashed
- 1/4 cup of aquafaba

Preparation:

1. In a food processor, combine the almond flour, coconut flour, whey protein, elf powder, xanthan gum, and mozzarella and pulse until the mixture resembles breadcrumbs.

2. Blend in the aquafaba until it forms a paste.

3. Cook for about 4 minutes, dividing the batter between two dash mini waffle plates (if only a small amount of steam comes out of the waffle iron).

4. Observations

5. Allow to cool for a few minutes before serving with the maple syrup.

6. You can use any flavor of whey protein isolate you want, but vanilla or quest cinnamon crunch are my favorites. Use unflavored whey protein and your favorite dressing (like 1/4 teaspoon of dressing for all but the bagel) to make a nice chaffle.

7. Pixie dust is made by grinding 20 grams of golden flaxseed, 10 grams of chia seeds, and 5 grams of psyllium husk powder in a spice or coffee grinder. This thickener can be used instead of or in addition to xanthan gum as a thickener.

8. The nutritional values are for a single serving.

Nutrition Facts: 130; Total Carbohydrates 4g; Net Carbohydrates 2g; Fat 8g; Protein 9g

KETOGENIC WHITE BREAD CHAFF | WONDER PAN CHAFFLE

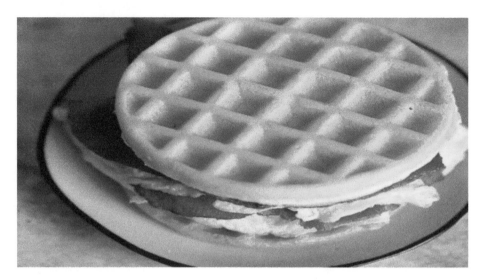

Time required: 10 min

Portions provided: 2

Ingredients:

- 1 egg
- 3 tablespoons of almond flour
- 1 tablespoon of mayonnaise
- 1/4 teaspoon baking powder
- 1 teaspoon of water

Preparation:

1. Preheat the waffle iron for mini waffles.
2. In a mixing bowl, whisk the egg until it is thoroughly combined.
3. Combine the almond flour, mayonnaise, yeast, and water in a mixing bowl.
4. After the waffle iron has heated up, carefully pour half of the batter into it and close the lid. Allow for 3-5 minutes of cooking time.
5. Remove the waffle iron carefully and set aside for 2-3 minutes to crisp.
6. For the second chaff, repeat the instructions.

Nutrition Facts: *Per serving*: Calories: 125; Total Fat 11.5g; Carbohydrates 2g; Net Carbohydrates g; Fibers g; Protein 5g

WAFFLE

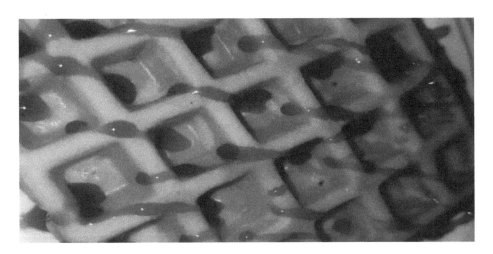

Time required: 5 min

Portions provided: 2

Ingredients:

- 2 cups of flour
- 1/2 cup of sugar
- 1 teaspoon of baking powder
- 1/2 teaspoon baking powder
- 1/4 cup oil
- 1 tablespoon of butter
- 2 eggs
- 1/2 cup milk with butter
- Pinch of salt

Preparation:

1. Combine all dry ingredients in a mixing bowl.
2. In a mixing bowl, crack the eggs and whisk in the grease, buttermilk, and butter until thoroughly combined.
3. Phase 2 of the waffle recipe is shown in this picture.
4. Mix in the dry ingredients until you have a smooth batter.
5. Butter your waffle iron and add the batter into it.
6. Chocolate syrup is a lot of fun.

VITA PODS

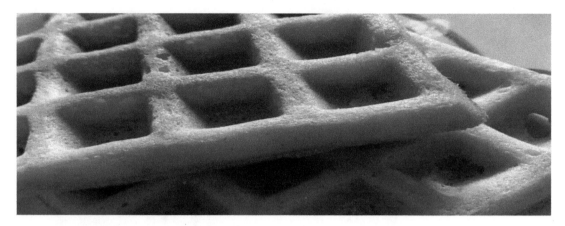

Time required: 5 min

Portions provided: 2

Ingredients:

- 1 cup half-life
- 1 cup of milk with butter
- 4 tablespoons butter, melted
- 2 eggs
- Pinch of salt
- 1/2 teaspoon baking powder
- Taste
- 1/2 teaspoon baking powder
- 2 tablespoons of sugar

Preparation:

1. Differentiate the yolks from the whites in a mixing bowl. And pound the whites until they're brittle
2. Combine the egg yolks, buttermilk, and butter in a mixing bowl; season with salt and pepper.
3. Allow the dry ingredients to soak before carefully folding in the beaten egg whites.
4. Cook the waffles in a preheated waffle iron.
5. Remove from the oven and serve hot, with fruit and a sweetener of your choosing, ice cream, whipped cream, or plain.

PODS 2

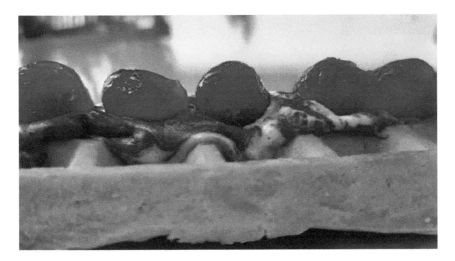

Time required: 5 min

Portions provided: 4

Ingredients:

- 2 cups of flour
- 3 tablespoons of sugar
- 2 eggs
- 11/2 cup of milk
- 1 tablespoon of flavor
- 1 teaspoon of baking powder
- 1/4 cup butter
- Pinch of salt

Preparation:

1. Waffle iron should be preheated.
2. Using an electric mixer, beat the eggs until frothy in a big mixing bowl.
3. In a separate cup, combine the flour, sugar, yeast, and salt.
4. In a mixing bowl, combine the buttermilk, eggs, vanilla extract, and melted butter.
5. Bake until golden brown in a preheated waffle iron.
6. Add your favorite toppings to finish.
7. Serve immediately.

PODS

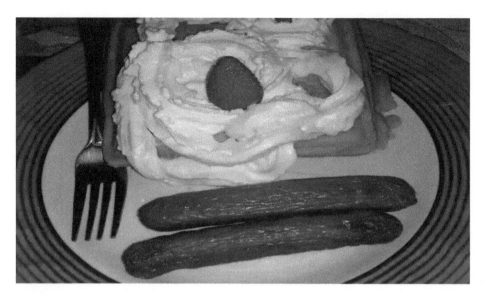

Time required: 30 min

Portions provided: 3

Ingredients:

- 2 cups of flour
- 2 tablespoons of sugar
- Pinch of salt
- 1 tablespoon of baking powder
- Half a cup of melted butter
- 1 teaspoon of vanilla flavor
- Half a cup of melted butter
- 1 3/4 cup buttermilk
- 2 eggs

Preparation:

1. Prepare your waffle iron by preheating it. In a mixing bowl, thoroughly combine all dry ingredients.

2. Stir in the beaten eggs, buttermilk, butter, and vanilla until all is well combined. Never give up. Knead the dough.

3. Fill the waffle iron halfway with batter and close it until golden brown. Serve with whatever you want, such as tea, coffee, whipped cream, or pancake syrup.

BEST BREAKFAST EVER

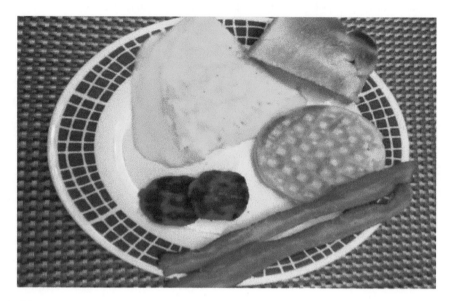

Time required: 30 min

Portions provided: 1

Ingredients:

- 1 whole egg
- Salt and pepper to taste)
- 1/2 cup of milk
- 3 slices of cheese
- 2 breakfast sausages (meatballs or mesh)
- 2 strips of bacon
- 2 slices of bread
- 1 waffle maker
- Syrup
- Butter

Preparation:

1. In a mug, whisk together the egg, salt, pepper, and milk. Pour the mixture into a skillet.

2. Place a slice of cheese on top. Then reverse your direction!

3. In a pan, brown the sausage on both sides.

4. Toast the waffle and toast together in the toaster oven. After that, butter the toast.

5. Cook the bacon in the microwave.

6. Enjoy your meal by serving it on a tray.

Preparation:

1. In a mug, whisk together the egg, salt, pepper, and milk. Pour the mixture into a skillet.

2. Place a slice of cheese on top. Then reverse your direction!

SUGAR FREE WAFFLES

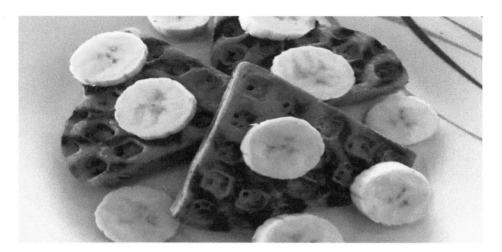

Time required: 10 min

Portions provided: 1

Ingredients:

- 1 egg
- 2 clear
- 1/2 ripe banana
- 1 tablespoon oatmeal
- 1 teaspoon cream cheese
- To taste cinnamon
- 1 pinch salt
- 1 tablespoon yeast
- Sweetener (optional)

Preparation:

1. Both of the ingredients should be mixed together.
2. Taste the mixture and add sugar, agave syrup, liquid saccharin, or other sweeteners if desired.
3. Create the cake in the oven or in a pan after greasing the mold. It takes no more than 10 minutes to complete.
4. The other half of the banana and a drizzle of agave syrup serve as toppings.

HEALTHY WAFFLES FOR BREAKFAST

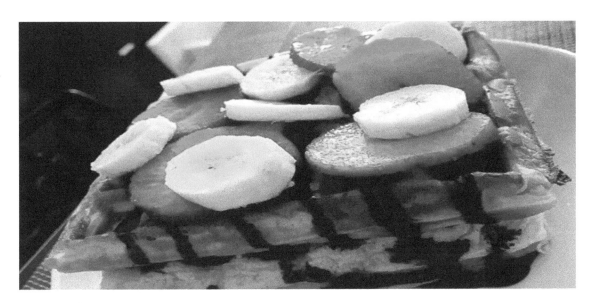

Time required: 30 min

Portions provided: 6

Ingredients:

- 80 gr oatmeal (used the normal one, but it can also be made with flavored flours)
- 1 yogurt 0% or 4 tablespoons of fresh cheese whipped 0%
- 1/2 banana
- 1 egg
- 3 clear
- 1 splash of vanilla essence
- 1 pinch salt
- 2 tablespoons yeast
- 1 dash of sweetener (optional)

Preparation:

1. Started by preheating the waffle maker. We choose the container in which the mixture will be prepared. We combine the egg, egg whites, yogurt or pounded fresh cheese, banana, and vanilla essence in a mixing bowl.

2. Whisk together the oatmeal, yeast, and a pinch of salt.

3. When the mixture has foamed up, pour it into the waffle maker in small batches, covering the gaps. My recommendation is that you put oil in the waffle iron and sweep it through it so that our delicious waffles do not stick.

4. Arrange the waffles on their respective plates and garnish them as desired! I used strawberries, bananas, and a 0% chocolate syrup. My father applied the honey touch, and it was fantastic!

CHAFFLES WITH ALMOND FLOUR

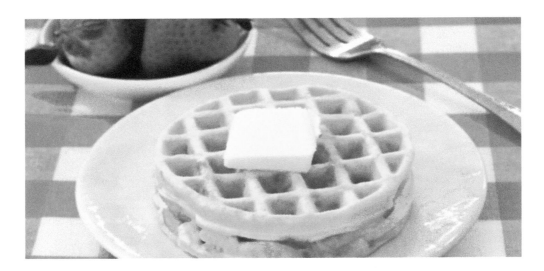

Time required: 20 min

Portions provided: 2

Ingredients:

- 1 large egg
- 1 tablespoon blanched almond flour
- ¼ teaspoon baking powder
- ½ cup shredded mozzarella cheese
- cooking spray

Preparation:

1. Combine the egg, almond flour, and baking powder in a mixing bowl. Put aside the batter after adding the mozzarella cheese.
2. Preheat a waffle iron as directed by the maker.
3. Coat the preheated waffle iron on both sides with cooking oil. Pour half of the batter into the waffle iron and spread it out with a spoon from the center. Close the waffle maker and cook for 3 minutes, or until the chaffle is finished to your liking. Remove the chaffle from the waffle iron with care and repeat with the remaining batter. Allow the chaffles to cool for 2 to 3 minutes before serving so that they crisp up.

Nutrition Facts: *Per Serving:* 132 Calories; Protein 10.8g; Carbohydrates 2g; Fat 9g; Cholesterol 111.1mg; Sodium 270.8mg.

KETO WAFFLES - LOW CARB / SUGAR FREE

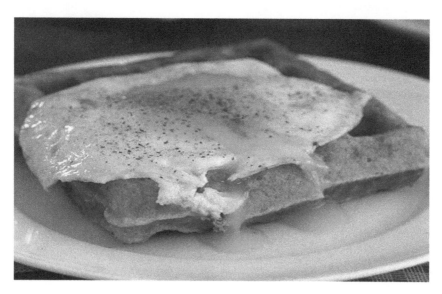

Time required: 25 min

Portions provided: 6

Ingredients:

- 3 large eggs (for extra fluffy waffles - separate the whites & whip until stiff peaks then fold into batter at the end)

- 2 tablespoons almond butter OR nut or seed butter of your choice

- 3 tablespoons granulated monk fruit sweetener , can also use SWERVE OR erythritol, add more if you prefer a sweeter waffle

- 2 tablespoons unsweetened almond milk

- 1/8 teaspoon apple cider vinegar , optional - helps give the waffles that fluffy buttermilk texture

- 1 teaspoon maple extract OR vanilla extract

- 1 cup superfine blanched almond flour

- 2 tablespoons coconut flour

- 1.5 teaspoons baking powder

- 1 teaspoon ground cinnamon , leave out if you prefer

Preparation:

1. Whisk together the eggs or egg yolks** in a big mixing bowl, then add the almond butter, sweetener, milk, apple cider (if using), and maple or vanilla extract.

2. Separate the yolks and whites first, then whip the whites until rigid peaks, then fold into the batter after adding the cinnamon.

3. Combine the almond flour, coconut flour, baking powder, and cinnamon in a large mixing bowl. Do not overmix. Mix until smooth and just mixed.

4. Permit the batter to thicken for 3-5 minutes while the waffle maker heats up. The baking powder would be able to activate as a result of this.

5. Spray the waffle maker with pure coconut oil spray and preheat it (or olive oil spray).

6. For mini waffles, use 1/4 cup batter; for Belgian waffles, use 2/3 cup batter. Cook, covered, until the waffle light turns orange (about 4-5 minutes depending on your waffle maker). Use a silicone spatula to flip the waffle over and cook for another round (another 4-5 minutes) until the light turns green for crispier waffles (recommended). Allow 15 seconds before transferring the crispy waffles to a tray.

7. Continue with the remaining batter. This recipe makes 6 (1/4 cup) Belgian waffles or 3 (2/3 cup) regular waffles.

8. Serve with whipped cream, melted butter, low-carb syrup, or fresh berries as toppings and sides.

POTATO WAFFLE WITH MELTED CHEESE AND EGG

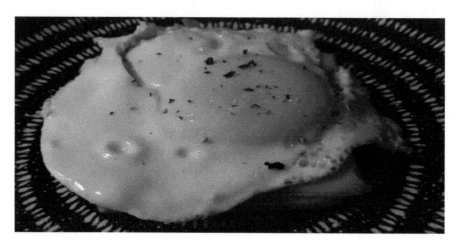

Time required: 10 min

Portions provided: 1

Ingredients:

- Potato waffle or waffle
- Cheese slices to melt
- Egg
- Fruit / juice / smoothie (recommended)
- Salt and pepper

Preparation:

1. Add the waffles after preheating the oven with the grill feature and turning them after 2 or 3 minutes, with the cheese already on top, and leaving them for another 2 or 3 minutes to melt the cheese.

2. In the meantime, we're preparing a fried egg.

3. Finally, we take the waffles out of the oven and cover them with the egg. Season to taste with salt and pepper, and you're done.

4. It's much richer with the yolk, and it doesn't curdle as much.

IBERIAN HAM AND CHEESE WAFFLES

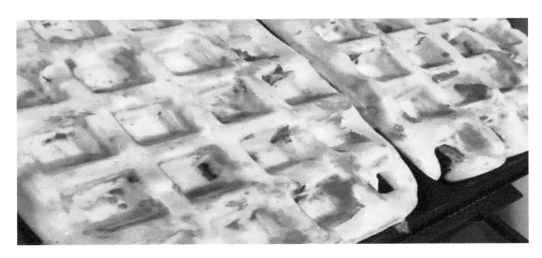

Time required: 20 min

Portions provided: 8

Ingredients:

- 2 eggs
- 1 cup milk
- 1 and 1/2 cup flour
- 15 gr baking powder (baking powder)
- 2 tablespoons butter
- Pinch salt and pepper
- Oregano
- 175 gr grated aged cheese
- 150 gr iberian ham
- Oil (if necessary to grease the waffle iron)

Preparation:

1. Started by preheating the waffle maker. We choose the container in which the mixture will be prepared. We combine the egg, egg whites, yogurt or pounded fresh cheese, banana, and vanilla essence in a mixing bowl.

2. Whisk together the oatmeal, yeast, and a pinch of salt.

3. We combine the flour and baking powder in a mixing bowl. It should be a semi-liquid, semi-thick mixture. Add a little more flour if it's too runny.

4. Finally, we add the ham and grated cheese.

5. Pour two scoops of the mixture into the waffle maker, which has been greased (it will depend on the waffle maker). We'll have our first waffles in about 2 minutes.

6. With these numbers, about 8 waffles are made.

VEGAN AND VEGETARIAN RECIPES

ZUCCHINI CHAFFLES

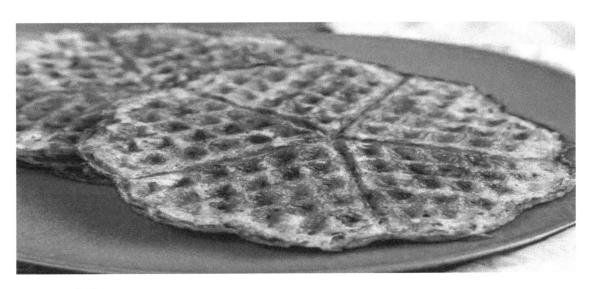

Time required: 5 min

Portions provided: 2

Ingredients:

- 1 cup Zucchini, grated
- 1 Eggs, beaten
- 1/2 cup shredded parmesan cheese
- 1/4 cup shredded mozzarella cheese
- 1 teaspoon Dried Basil, or 1/4 cup fresh basil, chopped
- 3/4 teaspoon Kosher Salt, divided
- 1/2 teaspoon Ground Black Pepper

Preparation:

1. Season the zucchini with 1/4 teaspoon salt and set aside as you gather your ingredients. Cover the zucchini in a paper towel and suck out any excess water just before using.

2. Beat the egg in a small bowl. Combine the grated zucchini, mozzarella, basil, 1/2 teaspoon salt, and pepper in a large mixing bowl.

3. Cover the bottom of the waffle iron with 1-2 tablespoons of shredded parmesan.

4. 1/4 of the zucchini mixture should be spread out. Close the lid and top with another 1-2 tablespoons of shredded parmesan. Use just enough to completely cover the surface. To learn how, watch the video.

5. Allow 4-8 minutes for the zucchini chaffle to cook, based on the scale of your waffle maker. When the chaffle no longer emits clouds of steam, it is almost done. Enable it to cook until it is well browned for the best performance.

6. Do not even overfill the container! In the Dash Mini, use no more than 1/4 cup of the chaffle mixture at a time.

7. These keep well in the freezer. To regain crispiness, freeze them and then reheat them in the toaster or air fryer.

8. These are great to eat on their own with butter or as a sandwich bread substitute.

Nutrition Facts: Calories 194; Carbohydrates 4g; Protein 16g; Fat 13g; Fiber 1g; Sugar 2g

KETO CAULIFLOWER CHAFFLES RECIPE

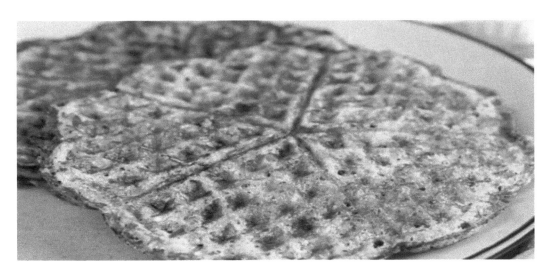

Time required: 9 min

Portions provided: 2

Ingredients:

- 1 cup riced cauliflower
- 1/4 teaspoon Garlic Powder
- 1/4 teaspoon Ground Black Pepper
- 1/2 teaspoon Italian Seasoning
- 1/4 teaspoon Kosher Salt
- 1/2 cup shredded mozzarella cheese, or shredded mexican blend cheese
- 1 Eggs
- 1/2 cup shredded parmesan cheese

Preparation:

1. In a mixer, combine all of the ingredients.
2. 1/8 cup parmesan cheese, grated into the waffle maker As seen in the video, make sure to cover the bottom of the waffle iron.
3. Pour the cauliflower mixture into the waffle maker.
4. On top of the mixture, add another sprinkling of parmesan cheese. Make sure the top of the waffle iron is covered.

5. You can make these in a mini waffle maker (I use the Mini Dash Waffle Maker), but you can also make them in a standard waffle maker.

6. These keep well in the freezer. Make a large batch and store it in the freezer for later.

HOW TO MAKE THE BEST CAULIFLOWER CHAFFLES EVER: TIPS AND TRICKS

1. Patience is needed. That is the most useful advice. They don't take long to make, but if you want a crisp keto waffle, you'll have to be patient and wait the 5-7 minutes it takes to crisp up. Just when you think you've got it figured out? Give it a minute or two more. Take your time.

2. Using several layers. On the top and bottom, don't skimp on the cheese. If you think you'll need more, go ahead and double the recipe. Crispiness comes from the crispy cheese on the bottom and top.

3. Waffles with a shallow depth. The shallower the waffle iron, the easier/faster it is to crisp up the chaffle if you want crispy waffles.

4. There should be no excess filling. Chaffle makers that are overfilled, well, they overflow. This results in a big mess! When in doubt, it's better to underfill rather than overfill. At a time, use no more than 1/4 cup of TOTAL ingredients.

5. There will be no peeking. Opening the waffle iron every 30 seconds just to check doesn't help the chaffle cook any quicker, I can tell you from a lot of personal experience. It's best not to open it for at least 4-5 minutes.

6. There will be no steaming. When using the Dash mini, the little blue light turns off when the chaffle is mostly cooked, but most importantly, the chaffle stops steaming as often. That's a clear indication that it's over.

7. It's time to get wet. If you wait until the waffle iron is hot before adding ingredients, they'll stick less and be easier to clean up.

8. It's a mat. So, let's talk about the overflow. It does seem to happen to me more often than I would like! Using a silicone trivet underneath the table has made cleanup a lot simpler for me.

9. Crispy Refreshment Allow for cooling before eating the chaffles. As they cool, they become crispier, so don't shove the hot chaffle into your mouth right away.

10. Make a couple of them. Make plenty to share; whether they're keto or not, everybody would want them.

Nutrition Facts: Calories 246; Carbohydrates 7g; Protein 20g; Fat 16g; Fiber 2g; Sugar 2g

KETO PARMESAN GARLIC CHAFFLES - 3 WAYS

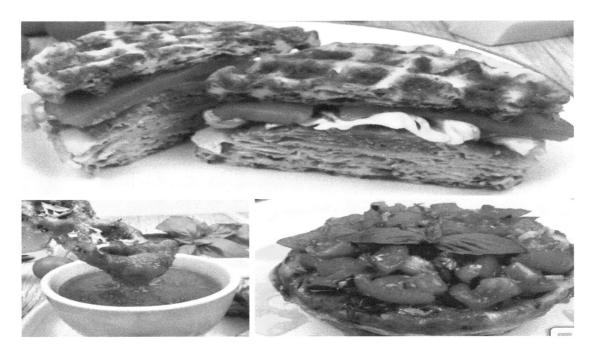

Time required: 6 min

Portions provided: 1

Ingredients:

- ½ cup shredded mozzarella cheese

- 1 whole egg, beaten

- ¼ cup grated Parmesan cheese

- 1 teaspoon Italian Seasoning

- ¼ teaspoon garlic powder

Preparation:

1. Start preparing the batter in your Waffle Maker (mine makes 4" waffles).

2. In a mixing bowl, whisk together all of the ingredients except the mozzarella cheese. Mix in the cheese until it is well mixed.

3. Apply nonstick spray (I used coconut oil) to your waffle plates and pour half of the batter into the middle. Cook for 3-5 minutes, depending on how crispy you want your Chaffles to be.

4. There are a few options for serving. Serve with a drizzle of olive oil, grated Parmesan cheese, and freshly chopped parsley or basil, for example.

NOTES ON THE RECIPE: 1. **Italian Chaffle Sandwich**

As directed above, make the base recipe. Add cold cuts, lettuce, and tomato you want. Ham, salami, lettuce, and roasted red pepper were included.

2. Breadsticks Chaffle

As directed above, make the base recipe. Cut each chaffle into four sticks and serve with Low Carb Marinara Sauce on the side.

3. Bruschetta de Chaffles

As directed above, make the base recipe. 3-4 chopped cherry tomatoes, 12 teaspoon chopped fresh basil, a drop of olive oil, and a sprinkle of salt Serve the chaffles with the sauce you made earlier

KETO TACO CHAFFLE (CRISPY TACO SHELLS)

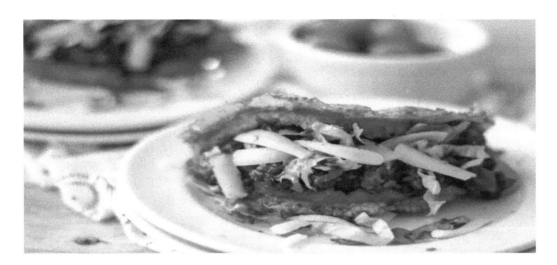

Time required: 8 min

Portions provided: 2

Ingredients:

- 1 egg white
- 1/4 cup Monterey jack cheese, shredded (packed tightly)
- 1/4 cup sharp cheddar cheese, shredded (packed tightly)
- 3/4 tsp water
- 1 tsp coconut flour
- 1/4 tsp baking powder
- 1/8 tsp chili powder
- pinch of salt

Preparation:

1. Once the Dash Mini Waffle Maker is heated, plug it in and lightly grease it.

2. In a mixing bowl, combine all of the ingredients and stir to combine.

3. Close the lid on the waffle maker after spooning out half of the batter. Set a timer for 4 minutes and don't open the lid before the timer goes off. It will seem that the taco chaffle shell isn't setting up properly if you do this, but it will. Before raising the lid, you must let it cook for the full 4 minutes.

4. Set the taco chaffle shell aside after removing it from the waffle iron. Repeat the procedure with the remaining chaffle batter.

5. To make a taco shell, flip a muffin pan over and place the taco chaffle shells between the cups. Allow a few minutes for the mixture to settle.

6. Remove from the oven and serve with the Best Taco Meat or your favorite taco recipe.

7. With your favorite toppings, enjoy this delicious keto crispy taco chaffle shell.

The nutritional information provided is only for the keto taco chaffle shells recipe.

Nutrition Facts: *Per Serving:* Calories 258; Carbohydrates 4g; Protein 18g; Fat 19g; Fiber 2g; Sugar 1g

KETO CHAFFLE GARLIC CHEESY BREAD STICKS

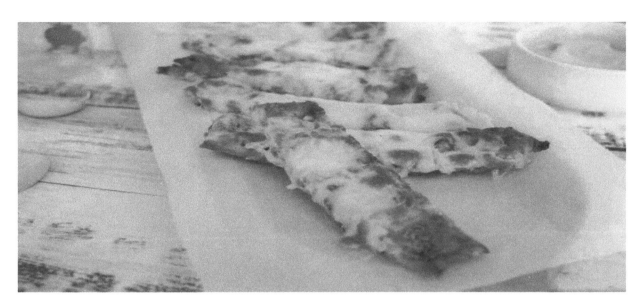

Time required: 10 min

Portions provided: 8

Ingredients:

- 1 medium egg
- ½ cup mozzarella cheese grated
- 2 tablespoons almond flour
- ½ teaspoon garlic powder
- ½ teaspoon oregano
- ½ teaspoon salt

For the topping:

- 2 tablespoons butter, unsalted softened
- ½ teaspoon garlic powder
- ¼ cup mozzarella cheese grated

Preparation:

1. Switch on your waffle maker and gently grease it (I spray it with olive oil). Beat the egg in a cup.

2. Mix in the mozzarella, almond flour, garlic powder, oregano, and salt until thoroughly combined.

3. Fill your waffle maker halfway with batter (my waffle maker is a square double waffle, so this mixture covers both waffle sections). Spoon half of the mixture into a smaller waffle maker at a time).

4. I spoon my batter into the waffle maker's center and gently spread it out to the edges.

5. Cook for 5 minutes with the lid closed.

6. Remove the cooked waffles with tongs and cut each waffle into four strips.

7. Pre-heat the grill and arrange the sticks on a plate.

8. Combine the butter and garlic powder, then scatter it over the sticks.

9. Place the mozzarella sticks under the grill for 2-3 minutes, or until the cheese has melted and is bubbling.

10. Eat right now! (Although we've eaten it warm, it's much better when it's made fresh.)

Nutrition Facts: *Per Serving*: 1 stick; Calories 74; Carbohydrates 0.9g; Protein 3.4g; Fat 6.5g; Fiber 0g

KETO EGGS BENEDICT

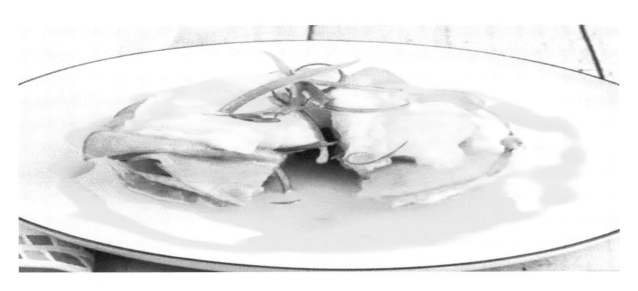

Time required: 30 min

Portions provided: 2

Ingredients:

- 2 egg whites
- 2 tbsp almond flour
- 1 tbsp sour cream
- 1/2 cup mozzarella cheese
- For the Hollandaise
- 1/2 cup salted butter
- 4 egg yolks
- 2 tbsp lemon juice
- For the Poached Eggs
- 2 eggs
- 1 tbsp white vinegar
- 3 ounces deli ham

Preparation:

1. To make the chaffle, whisk the egg white until it is frothy, then fold in the rest of the ingredients. Connect half of the chaffle mixture to the Dash Mini Waffle Maker and preheat it. Using nonstick cooking spray, coat the chaffle maker. Cook for approximately 7 minutes, or until golden brown. Repeat with the chaffle removed.

2. To make the Hollandaise sauce, follow these steps: Assemble a two-boiler system (a pot with a heat-safe bowl that fits on the top). Fill the pot with enough water to bring it to a boil, but not enough to cover the bottom of the dish.

3. Hollandaise sauce with a twist: In the oven, bring the butter to a boil. Toss the egg yolks into the double boiler's bowl and bring to a boil. While the pot is heating up, pour the hot butter into the tub.

4. Continuing with the Hollandaise, whisk quickly to warm the mixture from the water underneath the cup. Cook until the water in the pot has come to a boil, the egg yolk-butter mixture has thickened, and the mixture is very hot to the touch. Take the bowl out of the pot and squeeze in the lemon juice. Placed on the foot.

5. To poach an egg, fill your pot halfway with water (enough to fully cover an egg) and bring to a simmer. 2 tbsp white vinegar to 2 tbsp water Cook for 90 seconds after carefully dropping an egg into the simmering soup. Using a slotted spoon, remove the chicken.

6. To make the chaffle, toast it in the toaster for a few minutes. Half of the ham strips, one poached egg, and about 2 tablespoons of mayonnaise go on top of the crispy chaffle. Enjoy!

Nutrition Facts: *Per Serving: 1 chaffle eggs Benedict:* Calories 844; Carbohydrates 5g; Protein 32g; Fat 78g; Saturated Fat 41g; Cholesterol 728mg; Sodium 1220mg; Potassium 292mg; Fiber 1g; Sugar 2g; Vitamin A 2402IU; Vitamin C 6mg; Calcium 247mg; Iron 3mg; Net Carbohydrates 4g

Notes: Just 4 tablespoons of Hollandaise sauce are used in this recipe. There will be some left over. Refrigerate it and slowly warm it in a double boiler. If you microwave it, it will transform into scrambled eggs.

DAIRY-FREE AND EGG-FREE CHAFF BREAD RECIPE

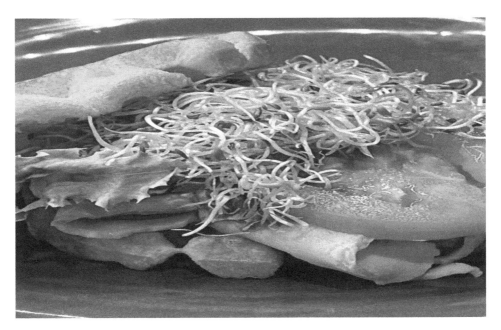

Time required: 3 min

Portions provided: 3

Ingredients:

- 3 tablespoons of almond flour
- 1 tablespoon of vegan sauce
- 1/8 teaspoon baking powder
- 1/4 cup egg juice an egg substitute

Preparation:

1. In a small mixing bowl, combine all of the ingredients and stir well until thoroughly combined.
2. Preheat the mini dash waffle iron and spoon half of the batter into it.
3. Allow for 3 minutes of simmering time.
4. Placed on a shelf to cool.
5. To make the second slice of bread, bake the last piece of dough.
6. This is ideal for low-carb sandwiches!

CREAM CHEESE CHAFFLE WITH LEMON CURD

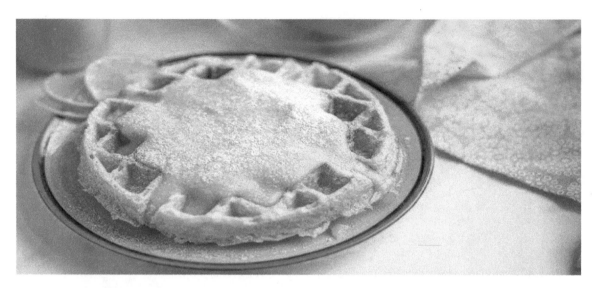

Time required: 49 min

Portions provided: 1

Ingredients:

- 1 batch keto lemon curd
- 3 large eggs
- 4 ounces cream cheese, softened
- 1 tablespoon low carb sweetener (I use Lakanto Monkfruit)
- 1 teaspoon vanilla extract
- 3/4 cup mozzarella cheese, shredded
- 3 tablespoons coconut flour
- 1 teaspoon baking powder
- 1/3 teaspoon salt

Preparation:

1. Prepare the lemon curd according to the package directions and chill until ready to use.

2. Meanwhile, preheat the waffle maker and oil it as normal.

3. Combine coconut flour, baking powder, and salt in a small mixing bowl. Set aside after thoroughly mixing.

4. Combine eggs, cream cheese, sweetener, and vanilla in a big mixing bowl. Beat with a hand mixer until frothy. It's fine if there are any cream cheese bits left over.

5. Continue beating the egg mixture with the mozzarella cheese.

6. Continue mixing the dry ingredients into the egg mixture until it is well mixed.

7. Pour the batter into a waffle maker that has been preheated and cook it like a waffle. Usually just a few minutes.

8. Pull waffles from waffle maker and serve with chilled lemon curd and optional whipped cream.

Nutrition Facts: *Per Serving:* Calories 302; Total Fat 24g; Saturated Fat 13g; Trans Fat 0g; Unsaturated Fat 9g; Cholesterol 246mg; Sodium 599mg; Carbohydrtates 6g; Net Carbohydrates 5g; Fiber 1g; Sugar 3g; Protein 15g

EVERYTHING BAGEL CHAFFLE WITH SMOKED SALMON CREAM CHEESE

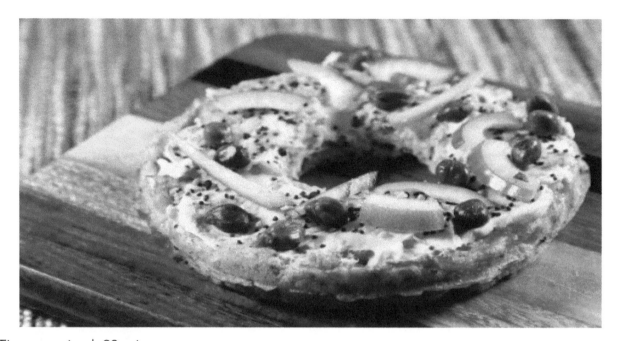

Time required: 20 min

Portions provided: 2

Ingredients:

- 1 large egg
- 3 teaspoons everything bagel seasoning, divided
- 1 teaspoon coconut flour
- ¼ teaspoon baking powder
- ½ cup shredded mozzarella cheese

For the topping:

- 4 tablespoons smoked salmon cream cheese spread (such as Philadelphia®)
- 1 teaspoon capers, drained
- 3 thin red onion slices

Preparation:

1. Pre - heat a waffle maker as directed by the manufacturer.

2. In a small mixing bowl, combine the egg, 2 teaspoons bagel seasoning, coconut flour, and baking powder. Add the mozzarella cheese and mix well.

3. Pour half of the batter into the waffle maker and spread it out with a spoon from the center. Close the waffle maker and cook for 3 to 4 minutes, or until the chaffle is finished to your liking and the waffle maker stops steaming.

4. Start by removing the chaffle from the waffle maker and put it on a rack to cool. Repeat with the remaining batter. Allow to cool for a few minutes to crisp up.

5. Distributed 1/2 of the salmon cream cheese on each chaffle and top with the remaining 1 teaspoon bagel seasoning, capers, and red onion. To make the chaffles look more authentic and enjoyable, cut out a circle in the middle with a sharp knife or a 1 1/2-inch round cookie cutter.

Nutrition Facts: *Per Serving:* Calories 232; Protein 12.5g; Carbohydrates 5.7g; Fat 15.3g; Cholesterol 141.1mg; Sodium 1013.7mg.

EASY CHAFFLE WITH KETO SAUSAGE GRAVY RECIPE

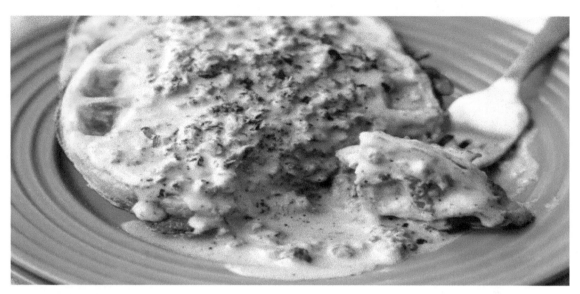

Time required: 10 min

Portions provided: 2

Ingredients:

- 1 egg
- 1/2 cup mozzarella cheese, grated
- 1 tsp coconut flour
- 1 tsp water
- 1/4 tsp baking powder
- pinch of salt
- For the Keto Sausage Gravy:
- 1/4 cup breakfast sausage, browned
- 3 tbsp chicken broth
- 2 tbsp heavy whipping cream
- 2 tsp cream cheese, softened
- dash garlic powder
- pepper to taste
- dash of onion powder (optional)

Preparation:

1. Enable to heat up by plugging the Dash Mini Waffle Maker into the wall. Cooking spray or a thin coating of grease is recommended.

2. In a small mixing cup, whisk together all of the ingredients for the chaffle.

3. Half of the chaffle batter should be poured into the waffle maker, closed, and cooked for about 4 minutes.

4. Remove the first chaffle from the waffle maker and produce the second chaffle in the same way. Crisp it up in the oven.

5. To make the Keto Sausage Gravy, combine all of the ingredients in a mixing bowl and whisk together

6. 1 pound breakfast sausage, cooked and drained. For this recipe, save 1/4 cup.

7. Make sausage patties with the remaining sausage and set aside 1/4 cup to brown for this recipe.

8. If you've never had breakfast sausage before, it's crumbled like ground beef.

9. Remove any excess grease from the skillet and add 1/4 cup browned breakfast sausage, along with the remaining ingredients, to the skillet. Bring to a boil, stirring constantly.

10. Reduce heat to medium and cook for another 5-7 minutes with the lid off, until the sauce thickens. If you'd like it very thick, you can add a bit of Xanthan Gum, but if you are patient with it simmering the keto sausage gravy will thicken. Then, it will thicken even more as it cools.

11. Combine salt and pepper to taste and spoon keto sausage gravy over chaffles.

Nutrition Facts: *Serving:* 1chaffle; Calories 212; Carbohydrates 3g; Protein 11g; Fat 17g; Saturated Fat 10g; Cholesterol 134mg; Sodium 350mg; Potassium 133mg; Fiber 1g; Sugar 1g; Vitamin A 595IU; Vitamin C 2mg; Calcium 191mg; Iron 1mg

VEGAN KETO CHAFFLE WAFFLE RECIPE

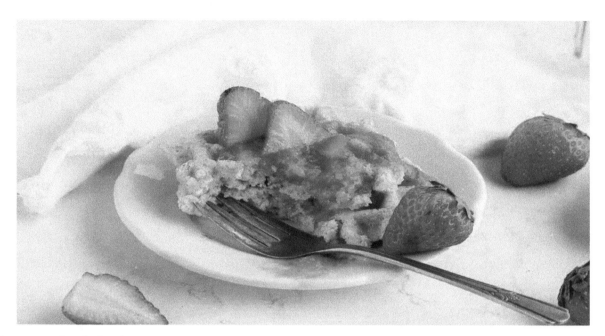

Time required: 6 min

Portions provided: 2

Ingredients:

- 1 tablespoon of flaxseed flour
- 2 tablespoons and a half of water
- ¼ cup low-carb vegan cheese
- 2 tablespoons of coconut flour
- 1 tablespoon of vegan, low-carb cream cheese, softened
- pinch of salt

Preparation:

1. Pre - heat the waffle iron to a medium-high temperature.

2. The second

3. In a small cup, combine the flaxseed flour and water. Allow 5 minutes for the mixture to thicken and become sticky.

4. To make the vegan chaff, whisk together all of the ingredients.

5. To make vegan keto waffles, combine all of the ingredients in a mixing bowl.

6. Pour the vegan waffle batter into the waffle iron's middle. Close the waffle iron and cook the waffle for 3-5 minutes, or until golden brown and strong. Pour half of the batter into a mini waffle iron if you're using one.

7. Fill the waffle iron halfway with the waffle batter.

8. Remove the waffle iron's vegan chaff and serve.

Nutrition Facts: Calories 114; Fat 7.3g; Protein 2.4g; Net Carbohydrates 5.5g

VEGAN CHAFFLE

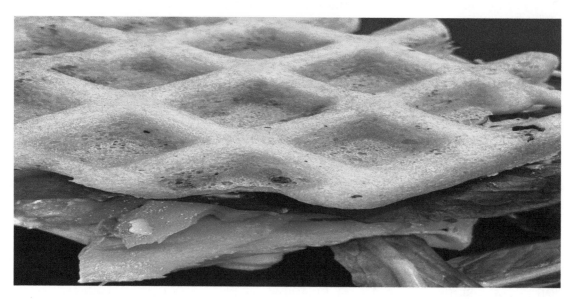

Time required: 5 min

Portions provided: 2

Ingredients:

- Rumford baking powder
- 3 tbsp Bob's red mill almond flour, super-fine
- Tbsp Spectrum light canola mayo, eggless, vegan
- Tbsp Just egg plant-based scramble

Preparation:

1. Mix and cook on a waffle maker.

Nutrition Facts: Calories 250 15%; Total Fat 17.65g 28%; Saturated Fat 0g 0%; Trans Fat 0g 0%; Cholesterol l0mg 0%; Sodium 291.55mg 13%; Potassium 135mg 3%; Total Carbohydrates 9.83g 4%; Dietary fiber 1.5g 6%; Sugars 1.5g 2%; Added sugars 0g 0%; Protein 12.65g 26%; Vitamin A 0mcg 0%; Vitamin C 0mg 0%; Calcium 55mg 6%; Iron 0mg 0%; Vitamin D 0mcg 0%

VEGAN WAFFLE WITH ICE CREAM

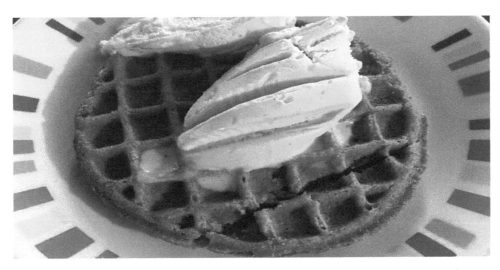

Time required: 5 min

Portions provided: 1

Ingredients:

- 2 scoops of vegetable vanilla ice cream
- 1-2 high protein waffles

Preparation:

1. Waffles that have been toasted
2. Enjoy your toasted waffle with a scoop of veggie ice cream!

ZUCCHINI, HAM AND CHEESE WAFFLES

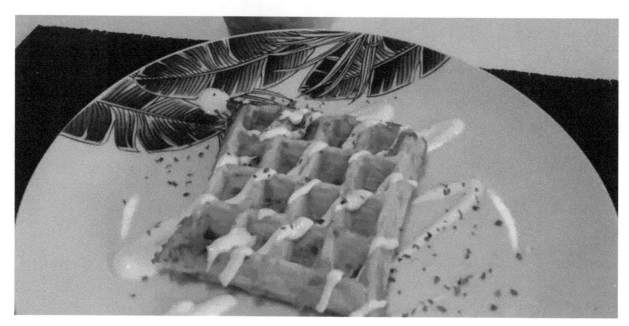

Time required: 1 h 1/2 min

Portions provided: 4

Ingredients:

- 300 gr flour
- 2 large zucchini
- 1/2 on royal yeast
- 4 slices serrano ham
- 150 gr grated or sliced cheese (to taste)
- Salt
- Pepper
- Milk (whatever you need)
- 4 eggs
- Yogurt sauce

Preparation:

1. Grate the zucchini and put it aside. In a mixing bowl, combine the flour, royal yeast, and milk (a little at a time) with the salt, pepper, and grated cheese, as well as the 4 beaten eggs. Mix the zucchini with the Serrano ham, which has been chopped very little, until a chubby mixture is formed.

2. Preheat the waffle maker after thoroughly mixing the ingredients. We used a saucepan to pour the batter into the waffle maker and spread it evenly. We shut it and leave it for 15 minutes (checking in on it from time to time). We placed on the plate with a little yogurt sauce on top to complement it, depending on the strength it needs.

CARROT CAKE WAFFLES

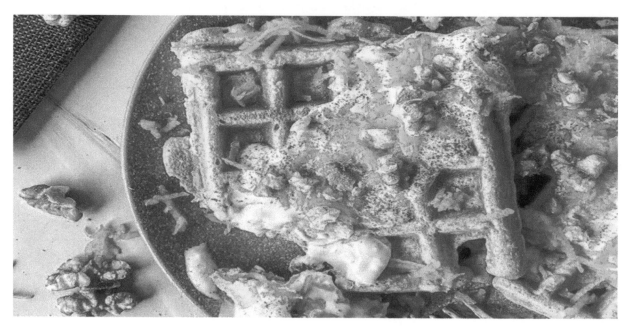

Time required: 10 minutes

Portion provided: 1

Ingredients:

- 1 egg
- 30 g neutral oatmeal
- 10 g coconut flour (or more oats)
- 1/2 tsp yeast
- 1/2 tsp cinnamon
- 1 pinch nutmeg
- 50 g grated carrot
- 1 tsp honey or agave syrup

For toppings:

- 40 g cream cheese spread
- 1 splash of milk
- 1/2 tsp honey or agave syrup
- A few drops of vanilla
- Additional features
- Walnuts
- Grated carrot

Preparation:

1. Thoroughly combine all waffle ingredients, brush the waffle maker with a little coconut oil, and pour the dough in when it is hot.
2. To make the topping, combine all of the ingredients, pour over the waffles, and top with chopped walnuts and crushed carrots.

HOMEMADE AND HEALTHY WAFFLES

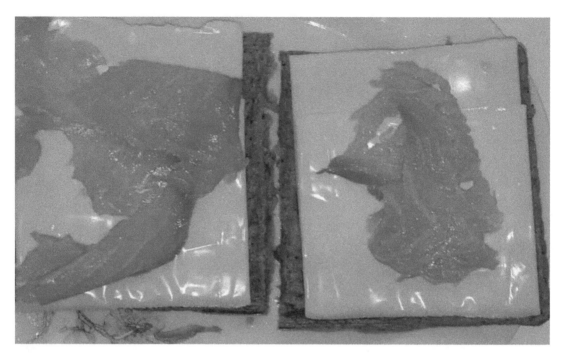

Time required: 15 min

Portions provided: 1

Ingredients:

- 25 gr oats
- 2 eggs
- 1 tablespoon yogurt beaten
- 1 pinch salt
- 1 pinch oregano
- 100 gr arugula
- 4 slices melted cheese
- 2 slices smoked salmon

Preparation:

1. Weigh 25 g of oatmeal and mix it with 2 eggs that have been pounded in a dish.

2. Also toss in some lamb's lettuce and arugula before removing all.

3. To give it flavor, we add salt, pepper, and oregano, and mix all together.

4. Preheat the waffle maker and apply the mixture after it has been beaten.

5. Place the waffles on a plate and top them with melting cheese and salmon until the mixture is ready (about 5 minutes in the waffle maker).

VEGETABLE WAFFLES AND SERRANO HAM (WAFFLES)

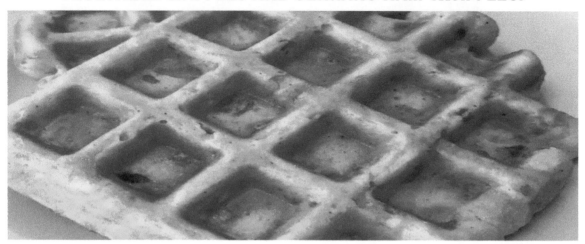

Time required: 40 min

Portion provided: 6-8

Ingredients:

- 1 medium onion
- 1 carrot
- 1 piece leek (10cm + -)
- 1 handful of mini Serrano ham taquitos
- 2 large eggs
- 115 gr flour
- 1 teaspoon baking powder
- 50 gr soft cheese grated by hand (or another that you like)
- 30 gr parmesan powder
- 40 ml whole milk (if you see that the dough is very hard, add a little more)
- Salt
- Pepper
- Garlic powder
- 1 tsp extra virgin olive oil (Evo)

Preparation:

1. Chopped the vegetables into very small pieces and fry them in evoo until they are tender. Salt, pepper, and garlic powder are used to season it. For around 10 minutes, we let it cool a bit

2. Combine the rice, yeast, eggs, milk, and cheeses in a mixing bowl and thoroughly combine. Season with a pinch of salt.

3. Combine the previously cooked vegetables with a handful of mini Serrano ham taquitos. We get along swimmingly.

4. Attach a small piece of dough to either side of the hot waffle maker without filling the entire square, which will expand and overflow. If you don't have a waffle maker, you can use a sandwich maker or a frying pan to cook them for about 5 minutes until golden brown.

SPINACH WAFFLES

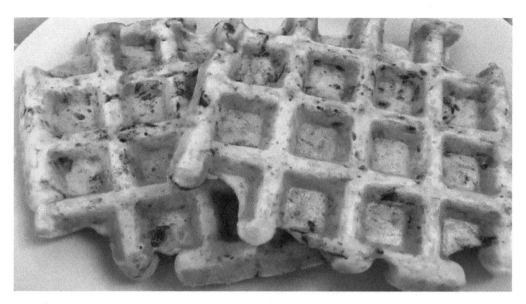

Time required: 20 min

Portions provided: 8

Ingredients:

- 4 cubes frozen spinach
- 2 large eggs
- 50 gr soft cheese grated by hand or another cheese that you like
- 30 gr parmesan powder
- 115 gr flour
- 1 teaspoon baking powder
- Garlic powder
- Salt
- Black pepper
- 40 ml whole milk

Preparation:

1. Defrost the spinach in a microwave-safe bowl with enough water to cover it for 3 minutes to cook it slightly, then drain the water, chop it up, and set aside

2. Combine the flour, yeast, and other ingredients in a separate cup.

3. Mix in the spinach, salt, pepper, and garlic powder until the mixture is fully homogeneous. You should taste it for salt and adjust accordingly.

4. A couple of tablespoons of batter on each side of the hot waffle maker (I have a 3-in-1 sandwich maker that works for everyone); not much that won't stick out later. We cook them for about 4 minutes inside to ensure a good browning.

5. Add anything to the top, like i did with Philadelphia and turkey, or we can leave them with nothing because they are already delicious! I hope you like it!

Notes: If you don't have a waffle maker, use a sandwich maker or a frying pan instead.

ZUCCHINI WAFFLES

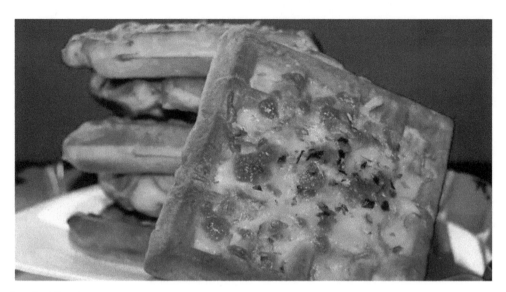

Time required: 10 min

Portions provided: 1

Ingredients:

- 1 large zucchini
- 1 egg
- 120 gr flour
- Salt and pepper
- Cheese for gratin (parmesan or mozzarella)
- Brush oil
- Oregano

Preparation:

1. Grate the zucchini and combine it with the egg and flour in a mixing bowl, seasoning it well.
2. Preheat the machine and oil the mold before filling it with 2 tablespoons of dough and sealing it.
3. The waffles are browned and set aside on kitchen paper.
4. Add the cheese and grill for a few minutes to see if the cheese has been gratinated. Remove from the oven and season with a pinch of oregano. Serve immediately. You're taking aim.
5. With this amount of batter, I was able to make 6 waffles.

ZUCCHINI WAFFLES WITH YOGURT SAUCE

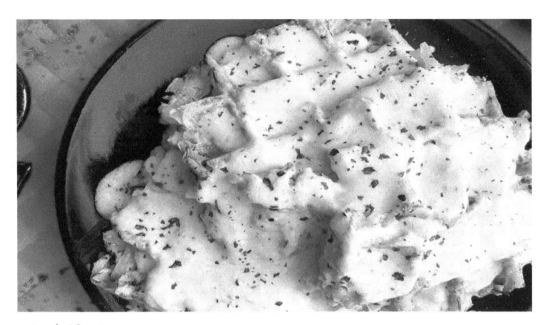

Time required: 10 min

Portions provided: 1

Ingredients:

- 1 zucchini (300g)
- 1/2 onion (optional)
- 1 egg
- 1 tbsp (30 g) whole wheat flour (spelled, oatmeal, wheat...)
- 1/2 tsp yeast
- Spices to taste (parsley, oregano, garlic powder...)

Optional:

- 20 g grated cheese (optional)

For the sauce:

- 125 g plain yogurt or smoothie fresh cheese
- 1 tbsp evo
- 1 splash of lemon juice
- To taste parsley

Preparation:

1. Grate the zucchini and onion and drain well with a cloth to eliminate any excess water.

2. Combine all of the ingredients in a mixing bowl until we have a dough.

3. We preheat the waffle maker and lightly grease it before making the waffles (i have made 3).

4. Combine all of the ingredients for the sauce, pour it over the pancakes, and that's it!

POTATO OMELETTE WAFFLES

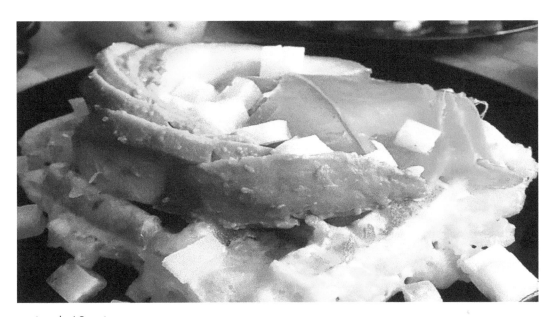

Time required: 10 min

Portions provided: 1-2

Ingredients:

- 220 g potato
- 30 g chopped onion
- 1 tsp extra virgin olive oil (Evo)
- 2 eggs
- 1/2 avocado
- 2 slices ham
- Cured cheese

Preparation:

1. Slice the potatoes thinly, combine with the Evo and onion, and cook for 7 minutes on high in the microwave.
2. Mix in the eggs with a fork until you have a lumpy consistency.
3. Preheat the waffle iron, grease it with coconut oil, pour in the batter, and cook until golden brown.
4. That's all there is to it! add our favorite toppings and call it a day!

CARROT CAKE FIT WAFFLES

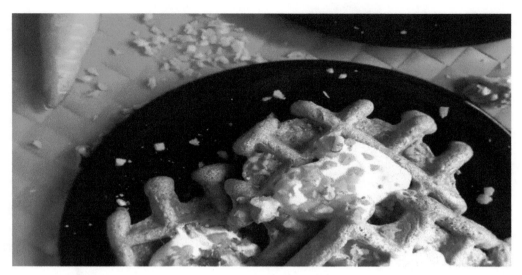

Time required: 10 min

Portions provided: 1

Ingredients:

- 100 g egg whites
- 30 g neutral oatmeal
- 25 g wholemeal spelled flour
- 1/2 tsp yeast (3g)
- 1/2 tsp cinnamon
- 1 pinch ginger
- 1 pinch nutmeg
- 1 carrot (75g)
- 1 tsp honey or agave syrup

For the topping:

- 40 g cheese spread
- 40 g fresh cheese whipped
- A few drops of vanilla
- 1 tsp agave syrup or honey
- 10 g walnuts

Preparation:

1. In a mixing bowl, combine the dry ingredients: oatmeal, spelled flour, yeast, cinnamon, ginger, and nutmeg.

2. Grate or crush the carrots, leaving a few tablespoons to garnish.

3. Beat the egg whites until stiff, then fold in the dry ingredients, carrot, and honey with enveloping movements until a homogeneous mass is formed.

4. Make the waffles by brushing a little coconut oil on the waffle iron and pouring a little batter in the middle (don't overdo it so it doesn't overflow).

5. To make the topping, combine the cheeses, honey, and vanilla extract; pour over the waffles; sprinkle chopped walnuts and crushed carrot on top; and that's all there is to it!

SPINACH WAFFLE

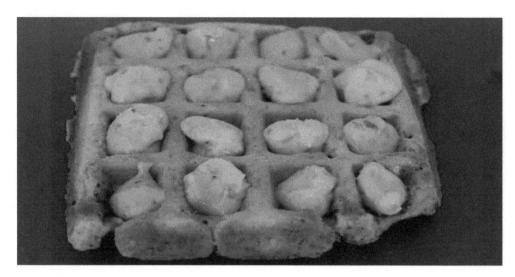

Time required: 20 min

Portions provided: 2

Ingredients:

- 3 eggs
- 300 ml milk
- 240 g flour
- 10g impeller
- 50 ml olive oil
- 1 avocado
- 100 g spinach
- 50 g grated parmesan
- Melted sheep cheese cream with boletus

Preparation:

1. To make the waffle dough, whisk together the eggs and milk in a blender glass. Using the impeller, add the flour and proceed to beat. When the dough is homogeneous, add the spinach, peeled avocado, lime zest, grated parmesan, and season to taste. Both of the ingredients should be thoroughly combined.

2. While the waffle iron is heating up.

3. Remove the waffles and set aside to cool. Fill the gaps in the waffles with a little cream on a plate.

SALTED FLAXSEED AND CHEESE WAFFLE

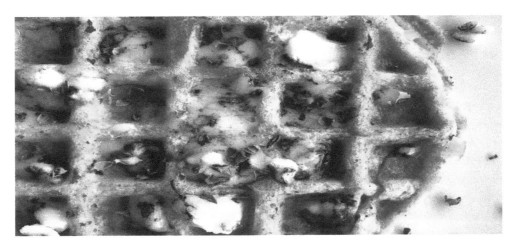

Time required: 25 min

Portions provided: 1

Ingredients:

- 1 egg
- 2 tablespoons ground flaxseed
- 1/2 baking powder
- 2 tablespoons grated mozzarella cheese
- Pinch salt

Preparation:

1. Combine all of the ingredients in a greased waffle maker. Serve according to personal preference.

WAFFLE FRIES WITH POTATOES

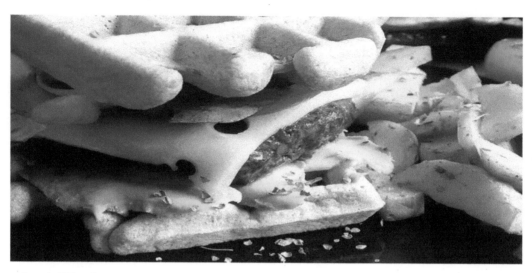

Time required: 25 min

Portions provided: 2

Ingredients:

- 1 egg

- 90 g clear

- 100 g wholemeal flour (wheat, spelled, oatmeal ...)

- 1/2 tsp baking powder

- Spices to taste (garlic and onion powder, oregano ...)

- Stuffed

- 2 hamburgers (beef, foal, veal ...)

- 2 slices cheese (I have used Emmental)

- Lettuce leaves

- 1 medium tomato

- 1/2 avocado

- Potatoes

- 1 medium potato

- Spices to taste (garlic and onion powder, oregano, paprika ...

Preparation:

2. Thoroughly combine all waffle ingredients and cook them in the waffle maker (heat it, brush with coconut oil and let it cook for a couple of minutes until ready).

3. When we turn the hamburgers over on the grill, we put a slice of cheese on top so that it melts.

4. Use the bread waffles to assemble the burgers with the rest of the ingredients, and that's it!

5. Cut the potato into sticks and mix it with the spices before placing it in the microwave for 4 minutes at 800w (in a lékué steam case) and serving it with our waffle-burgers.

ZUCCHINI WAFFLES STUFFED WITH MOZZARELLA

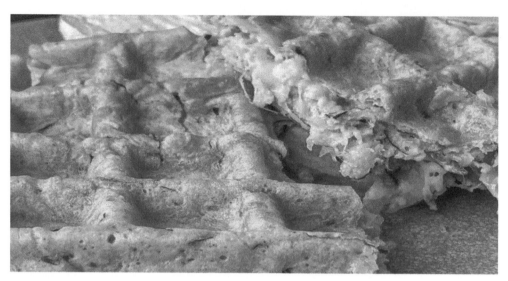

Time required: 10 min

Portions provided: 2

Ingredients:

- 100 g zucchini grated and drained
- 60 g oatmeal (or other whole grain)
- 2 eggs
- To taste garlic and onion powder
- 1/2 tsp yeast
- 2 slices fresh mozzarella

Preparation:

1. Grate the zucchini and rinse it with a clean rag.
2. You thoroughly combine all of the ingredients until we have a homogeneous mixture.
3. Part of the dough is poured into the waffle maker (which has been preheated and greased with coconut oil), followed by a slice of mozzarella and more dough.
4. Cook it for a few minutes before it's done and ready to eat!

JICAMA LOADED BAKED POTATO CHAFFLE

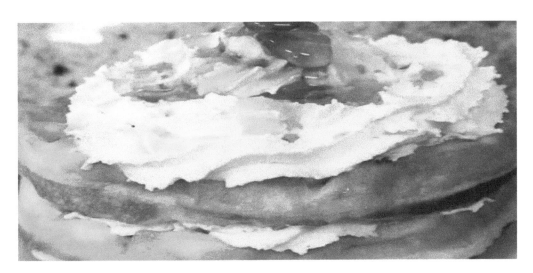

Time required: 30 min

Portions provided: 4

Ingredients:

- 1 large jicama root
- 1/2 medium onion, minced
- 2 garlic cloves, pressed
- 1 cup cheese of choice (I used Halloumi)
- 2 eggs, whisked
- Salt and Pepper

Preparation:

1. Jicama should be peeled and shredded in a food processor.

2. In a big colander, shred the jicama and season with 1-2 teaspoons of salt. Enable to drain after thoroughly mixing.

3. Squeeze as much liquid out as you can (very important step)

4. 5-8 minutes in the microwave

5. Combine all ingredients in a mixing bowl.

6. Spray a little cheese on the waffle iron before adding 3 T of the mixture, then top with a little more cheese.

7. 5 minutes in the oven Cook for another 2 minutes on the other hand.

8. Add a dollop of sour cream, bacon, cheese, and chives to the top!

Nutrition Facts: Calories 168; Total Carbohydrates 5.1g; Net Carbohydrates 3.4g; Fat 11.8g; Fiber 1.7g; Sugar 1.2g; Protein 10g

What exactly is a jicama? Jicama root is a Mexican round root vegetable with a texture close to that of a potato. It has a low calorie count but is rich in essential nutrients. Per 100g of jicama, there are around 5 net carbs. Fiber, vitamin C, and potassium abound in jicama! Insoluble fiber is also present.

If you haven't tried jicama yet, you have nothing to lose — and if you're looking to lose weight, this may be your new favorite.

SWEET AND SAVORY RECIPES

SAVORY PEPPER, YORK HAM AND MOZZARELLA WAFFLES

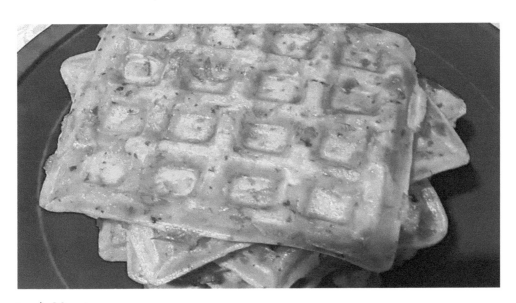

Time required: 30 min

Portions provided: 8

Ingredients:

- 200 ml milk
- 2 eggs
- 60 g grated cheese
- 200 g flour
- 2 teaspoons baking powder
- 150 g ham in small cubes
- 150 g red pepper, small dice
- Olive oil
- To taste paprika
- Salt taste
- To taste pepper

Preparation:

1. We whisked the eggs, milk, and cheese together.

2. Combine the rice, yeast, paprika, salt, and pepper in a mixing bowl.

3. All is beaten until there are no lumps.

4. In a frying pan, sauté the peppers and sweet ham with a pinch of salt and a drizzle of oil.

5. Add to the mix and thoroughly combine everything.

6. Pour a level scoop of the mixture into the waffle maker (I use an ice cream scoop scoop) and cook until the green pilot light in the waffle maker lights up or they are golden brown to taste.

PEPPER WAFFLES WITH POACHED EGG

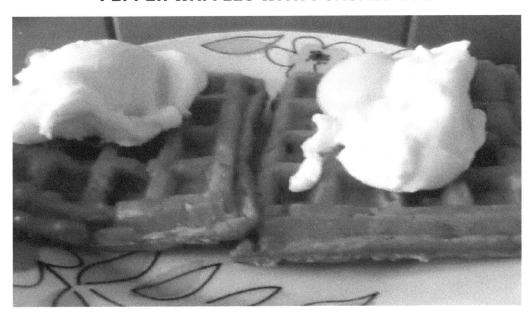

Time required: 15 min

Portions provided: 7

Ingredients:

- 1 red bell pepper
- 1 green pepper
- 1 yellow bell pepper
- 100 gr wheat flour
- 150 gr cornstarch
- 100 gr grated cheese
- Salt
- Ground black pepper
- 1 teaspoon sweet paprika
- 2 tablespoons baking powder
- 1/2 teaspoon baking soda
- 1 egg
- 60 ml olive oil
- 300 ml milk

Preparation:

1. Peppers should be washed and diced before being fried in a pan with a little oil.

2. In a mixing bowl, whisk together the egg, milk, and 60 ml oil; stir in the sifted flours, yeast, and bicarbonate. Season to taste with salt and pepper, then stir in the sweet paprika, sautéed peppers, and grated cheese.

3. Wait for the batter to cool before pouring it into the waffle iron.

4. Pour water into a saucepan and bring to a boil with a splash of vinegar, then crack an egg into a cup. With the aid of a spoon, bring the water to a boil and stir to create a whirlpool.

5. Cook for 4 to 6 minutes after carefully adding the egg. After that, move it to a plate lined with absorbent material.

6. Serve each waffle with a poached egg and enjoy!

SAVORY WAFFLES WITH MOZZARELLA CHEESE AND PARMESAN CHEESE

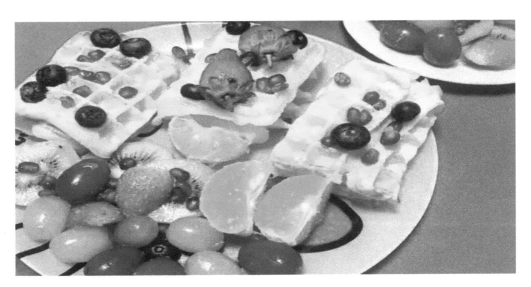

Time required: 25 min

Portions provided: 2

Ingredients:

- 2 cups flour (prepared)
- 2 tbsp butter or (lard)
- 1 egg
- 1/2 cup mozzarella cheese
- 1/2 cup parmesan cheese
- 1/2 cup fresh milk calculate
- To taste salt

Optional:

- Chantilly, white delicacy, chocolate fugde

Preparation:

1. Mix the two cheeses, egg, butter, milk, flour, and salt for 3 minutes, making sure everything is well combined. Let the dough rest in the fridge for 10 minutes.

2. Heat the waffle iron, but not before brushing it with butter or oil and removing the excess.

3. Allow the waffle iron to cool before covering it. Cover and wait for it to cook.

4. Remove it until it's done and repeat until we've finished all of the dough. Spread jam on it, roll it up, and serve it with a variety of fruits.

FLOURLESS POTATO, CHEESE AND ONION WAFFLES

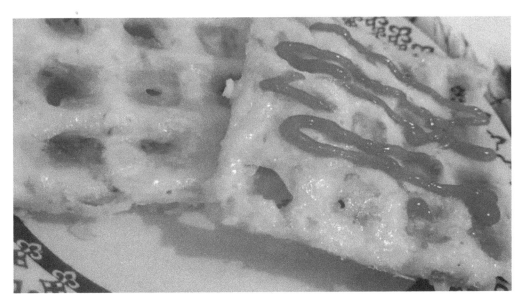

Time required: 30 min

Portions provided: 2

Ingredients:

- 3 medium potatoes
- 1 large onion
- 1 clove garlic
- 3 eggs
- 50 gr. Reggian cheese
- Salt and pepper to taste
- Oil for sautéing and brushing

Preparation:

1. Wash the potatoes well with a brush and cook them from cold water for 15 minutes (or 3 minutes on each side in the microwave) (or 3 minutes on each side in the microwave). They have to be cooked but firm in the center. We grate them with a coarse grater after they've been cooked and cooled (with the shell and all).

2. Chop the onion and garlic, then brown them in a frying pan with a little oil. Allow to cool.

3. In a mixing bowl, gently beat the eggs with salt and pepper, then add the reggian cheese, garlic, onion, and grated potatoes that have already been grated. Combine thoroughly.

4. Waffle iron should be plugged in. Use it in accordance with their model. When the oven is hot, brush the plates with neutral oil and fill each mold with around 2 or 3 tablespoons of the preparation. Cook for 5-10 minutes, or until the waffles are golden brown, after closing the waffle iron. Using a spatula, carefully remove them.

SAVORY KETO WAFFLES WITH CHICKEN AND CHEESE

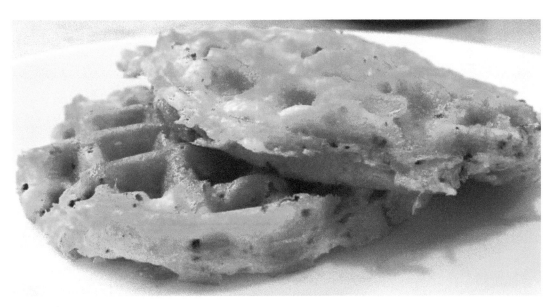

Time required: 30 min

Portions provided: 6

Ingredients:

- 1/2 cup almond flour
- 1 TBS psillyum husk
- 4 eggs
- 1/2 cup heavy whipping cream
- Pinch of salt
- 1 tsp baking powder
- 1 cup shredded cheese like Monterey Jack or gouda
- 1 cup of chicken leftovers and ham cut into small pieces
- Pepper and herbs of your choice

Preparation:

1. In a large mixing bowl, whisk together almond flour, psyllium husks, baking powder, salt, eggs, and heavy whipping cream until smooth.

2. Stir in the shredded cheese, ham, and chicken meat, which has been cut into small bits, with a fork.

3. Set aside the mixture for 5 minutes.

4. Use a waffle iron or a frying pan to produce waffles.

5. If you're using a frying pan, use butter or ghee to cook it in.

6. Serve with a cup of yogurt and waffles.

7. Serve with a dollop of cream cheese or butter on top; it'll be great!

Nutrition Facts: *for 1 waffle:* Calories 230; Carbohydrates 1.5 g; Fat 20 g; Protein 12 g.

CHEESY SAUSAGE WAFFLE

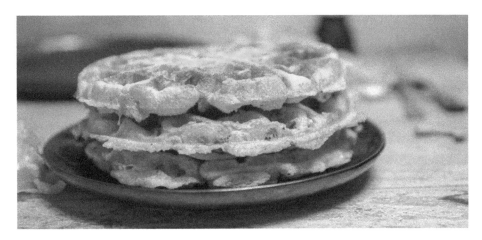

Time required: 25 min

Portions provided: 2

Ingredients:

- 3 thick sausages
- 80 g butter plus extra to serve
- 80 g almond meal
- 90 g whey protein isolate*
- 60 g cream cheese
- 80 g cheddar cheese small cubes
- 120 g thickened cream
- 100 g sour cream
- 1 egg
- 1 teaspoon baking powder
- 1 teaspoon baking soda
- 2 teaspoons xanthan gum

Preparation:

PROCESS USED IN THE PAST

1. Squeeze small sausage meatballs from the sausage skin. Fry until cooked through in a fry pan over medium high heat. Make a reservation.
2. 1 minute on the stove or in the microwave to melt butter
3. Mix the remaining ingredients in a mixer fitted with a dough hook or in a food processor until thoroughly mixed. Mix in the sausage meatballs.
4. Cook in a waffle iron that has been preheated and buttered according to the manufacturer's instructions. Serve with a dollop of butter and a slice of avocado on top.

THERMOMIX METHOD

1. Try squeezing small sausage meatballs from the sausage skin. Fry until cooked through in a fry pan over medium high heat. Make a reservation.
2. 3 minutes at 80°C/speed 1 to melt butter
3. Mix in the remaining ingredients for 3 minutes on the dough setting. Mix in the sausage meatballs.
4. Cook in a waffle iron that has been preheated and buttered according to the manufacturer's instructions. Serve with a dollop of butter and a slice of avocado on top.

Nutrition Facts: *Per Serving:* Calories 25; Carbohydrates 2g; Protein 7g; Fat 23g; Saturated Fat 11g; Cholesterol 73mg; Sodium 362mg; Potassium 124mg; Fiber 1g; Sugar 0g; Vitamin A 535IU; Vitamin C 0.2mg; Calcium 103mg; Iron 0.6mg

Notes: One waffle wedge equals one serving. You may raise the serving size while keeping the carb count low. The portions are remarkably substantial.

Replace the sausages with mushrooms for a vegetarian option: jalapenos, artichokes, or tomato and green onions are all good options.

Waffles can be stored in the freezer.

Sunflower seed meal is a nut-free substitute.

The batter is really stiff.

KETO WAFFLES STUFFED WITH CREAM CHEESE

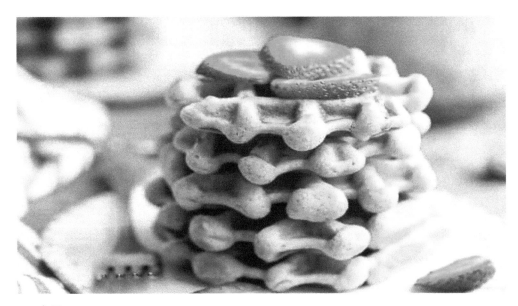

Time required: 7 min

Portions provided: 4

Ingredients:

- 1 teaspoon cooking oil
- 4 eggs large
- 4 tablespoons mayonnaise
- 1 tablespoon almond flour
- 2 tablespoons cream cheese

Preparation:

1. Cooking oil should be applied to the waffle iron's surface. To use the iron, turn it on to heat it up.

2. With a hand mixer or blender, combine the eggs, mayonnaise, and almond flour until smooth.

3. Cream cheese should be cut into 1x1 centimeter cubes.

4. Pour the batter into the hot waffle iron's middle. Before pushing the lid down, spread a quarter of the cream cheese bits in the iron wells.

5. Close the lid and start cooking the waffle until the cream cheese has been distributed. As the batter cooks, steam can escape from the waffle iron's seal; this is natural, but be careful of the hot steam!

6. Cook for 3-5 minutes, or until golden brown on top.

7. Take the waffle from the iron and place it on a tray. Serve plain or with a low-carb topping of your choice.

Nutrition Facts: Calories 201; Carbohydrates 1g; Protein 6g; Fat 19g; Saturated Fat 4g; Cholesterol; 177mg; Sodium 174mg; Potassium 70mg; Vitamin A 335IU; Calcium 35mg; Iron 0.8mg

BROCCOLI & CHEDDAR KETO WAFFLES

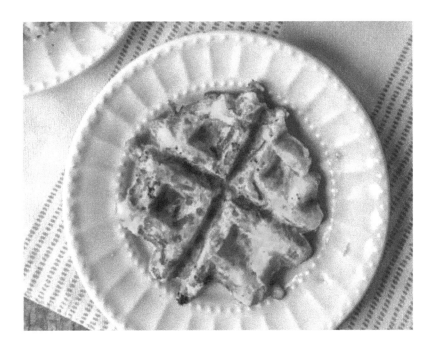

Time required: 10 min

Portions provided: 1

Ingredients:

- ⅓ cup raw broccoli, finely chopped 20g
- ¼ cup cheddar cheese, shredded 28g
- 1 egg
- ½ tsp garlic powder
- ½ tsp dried minced onion
- salt and pepper, to taste
- cooking spray

Preparation:

1. Warm up your waffle iron by plugging it in.

2. Crack the egg in a small bowl and pound it with a fork.

3. Combine the broccoli, cheese, garlic powder, onion, salt, and pepper in a large mixing bowl.

4. Spray the waffle iron with cooking spray (if necessary) and pour in the egg mixture. Close the waffle iron and cook until the light turns off, signaling that one cycle has completed.

5. Close the lid once more and cook for another period.

6. With tongs or a fork, carefully remove the waffles from the waffle iron when finished.

7. Have fun! Or butter, sour cream, or ranch dressing on the side.

Nutrition Facts: *Per Serving:* Calories 125; Carbohydrates 4g; Protein 7g; Fat 9g; Fiber 1g

BANANA WAFFLES

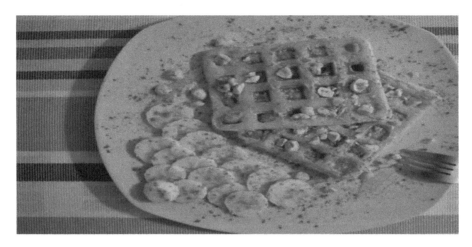

Time required: 5 minutes

Portions provided: 1

Ingredients:

- 2 clear
- 2 tablespoons whole oat flour
- 1/2 banana
- 1 tablespoon quark cheese
- Jet agave syrup
- Cinnamon

Preparation:

1. For a few seconds, beat all of the ingredients together until a homogeneous, lump-free dough forms.

2. That's it for the waffle maker. It's even possible to transform it into pancakes.

WAFFLES FIT GOLDEN

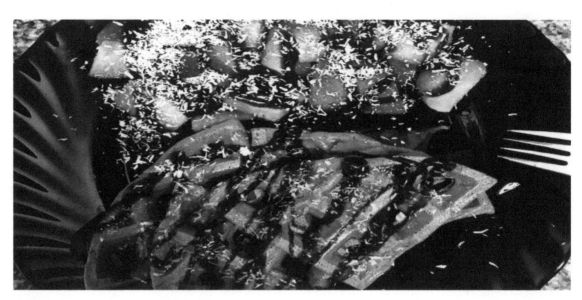

Time required: 20 min

Portions provided: 1-2

Ingredients:

- 40 gr wholemeal oatmeal
- 3 clear
- 1 tablespoon of 100% cocoa
- 1 dessert spoon of olive or coconut oil
- 1 tablespoon cream cheese 0%
- 1 dessert spoon of panela (optional) or another sweetener if we want

Preparation:

1. In a mixing bowl, combine all of the ingredients and beat until smooth.
2. While the mixture rests for 3 minutes, preheat the waffle maker.
3. Pour the batter into the waffle iron and "bake" until the waffles are large and golden.

CRISPY CHEESE WAFFLES

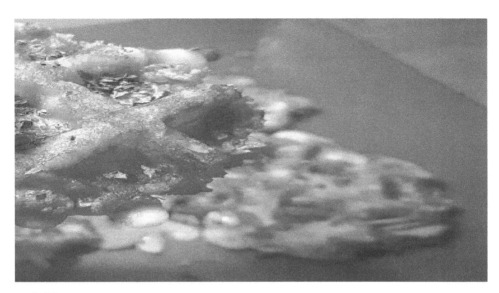

Time required: 20 min

Portions provided: 1/2

Ingredients:

- 150 g mozzarella in taco
- 40 g whole wheat flour
- 40 g corn flakes s / a 1 egg

Preparation:

1. Corn flakes are crushed into very small bits.
2. The flour, beaten egg, and corn flakes are divided into three bowls.
3. The mozzarella was sliced into squares of the same size.
4. The waffle maker is greased and preheated.
5. Batter (flour, egg, and corn flakes)
6. Place each piece in the waffle iron's center and cook for a few minutes, or until golden brown (do not take them out ahead of time or they will stick)
7. Take it out and season it to taste.

EASY CROFFLES (CROSSAINTS IN WAFFLE IRON)

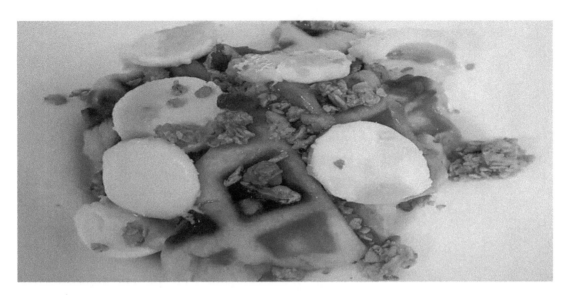

Time required: 40 min

Portions provided: 3

Ingredients:

- Pillsbury crescents rolls
- Nuts

Preparation:

1. Set the crescents aside after unrolling them. Crushes a handful of almonds, granola, or cheese.

2. Fill each crescent with your favorite nuts, cheese, or even sausage before rolling it up. To fluff them up, roll them up and bake for just 3 minutes. Remove them from the oven and place the crescents on a hot, buttered waffle iron. Let them out when they're done cooking and you're done! Croquettes

3. Serve with a variety of toppings. Granola, maple syrup, and cheese were among the items requested by the children.

ALMOND AND BANANA WAFFLES

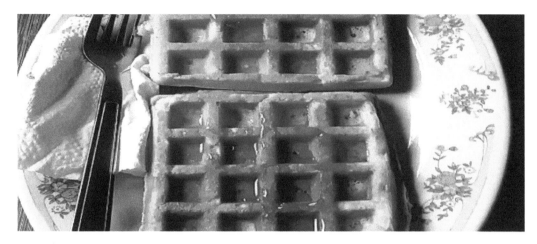

Time required: 15 min

Portions provided: 2

Ingredients:

- 1 cup of almond flour
- 2 ripe banana puree
- 2 eggs beaten
- 2 teaspoons baking powder
- 2 tablespoons of honey
- 1/2 cup milk/coconut milk

Preparation:

1. Make a bun out of your dry ingredients.
2. Mix in the wet ingredients gently.
3. Cook your waffles in a hot waffle iron.
4. Serve with a drizzle of honey on top.

FRIED WAFFLES

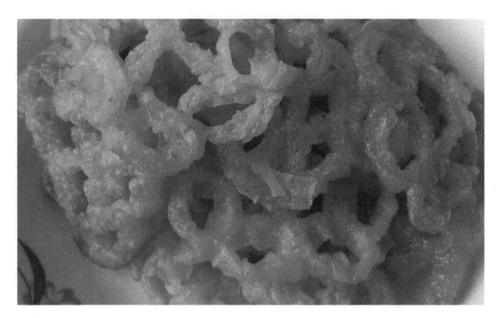

Time required: 30 min

Portions provided: 4

Ingredients:

- 2 cups of flour
- 1/2 cup of sugar
- 1/2 teaspoon of baking powder
- Water
- Fry oil
- Tool for roasting waffles

Preparation:

1. In a mixing bowl, combine the flour, baking powder, and salt.
2. Mix in the sugar and baking soda.
3. To make a runny dough, gradually add the water.
4. To reheat the waffle iron, heat the oil and place it in it.
5. Please put it in the dough to stitch some pasta when it is hot, then return it to the oil when it is hot. After removing the waffle from the waffle iron, it is fried until golden brown.

WAFFLES WITH HAM AND CHEESE

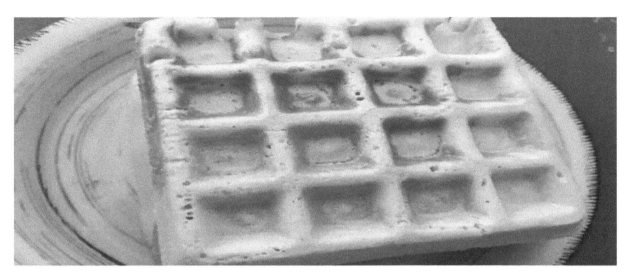

Time required: 30 min

Portions provided: 4

Ingredients:

- 1 1/2 cup commercial pancake flour
- C / n butter
- 2 slices thin leg ham
- 2 slices manchego cheese, gouda, chihuahua
- C / n mustard
- C / n aioli or mayonnaise

Preparation:

1. Follow the manufacturer's instructions for making the batter.
2. Spread butter on the waffle iron and heat it up. Pour enough batter to fully cover it.
3. Spread mustard on one side and aioli or mayonnaise on the other.
4. One of them put the ham in the oak, and the other put the cheese in the other.
5. Good luck with your meal.

WAFFLES FIT IN THE OVEN

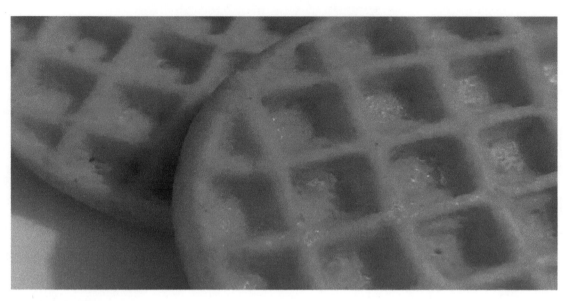

Time required: 10 min

Portions provided: 2

Ingredients:

- 4 tablespoons whipped cheese 0%
- 80 gr oatmeal
- 4 egg whites
- 1 teaspoon vanilla essence
- 1 teaspoon and a half yeast
- You can add some kind of sweetener

Preparation:

1. To begin, whisk together the egg whites and beaten cheese. An egg and its white can also be used. We combine the sifted flour and yeast in a mixing bowl. And there's vanilla.

2. Honey, sweetener, or brown sugar may be used as a sweetener. I like to leave it out and then cover it with sweet toppings like jam, sugar, hazelnut cream, cinnamon, or baked apple.

3. We put the mixture in a greased baking dish (depending on the mold, you might need more mixture). Preheat the oven to 170° F and bake for about 15 minutes.

4. They're fluffy waffles with a lot of flavor. If you want a crunchy texture, I've read that removing them when they're almost done and bathing them in sugar before putting them back in the oven is the trick.

5. If you don't want to use sweeteners or vanilla, apply a pinch of salt and eat them with crispy toppings.

OATMEAL FITNESS WAFFLES

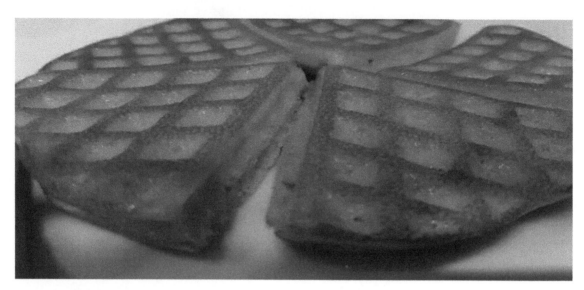

Time required: 25 min

Portions provided: 3-4

Ingredients:

- 180 ml egg white
- 60 gr oat flour (cookie flavor in my case)
- 4 tablespoons fresh whipped cheese 0%
- 7 gr baking powder
- Sweetener (optional)

Preparation:

1. In a blender glass, thoroughly combine all of the ingredients.
2. Preheat the oven to 200 degrees as we prepare the mixture.
3. Place the mixture in the molds and place them in the oven once the oven is hot.
4. Allow 15-20 minutes for baking, depending on the oven, and check with a toothpick to ensure it is not sticky.
5. They'd be prepared.
6. To taste, garnish with marmalade or sugar-free syrups.

POTATO WAFFLES WITH SMOKED SALMON

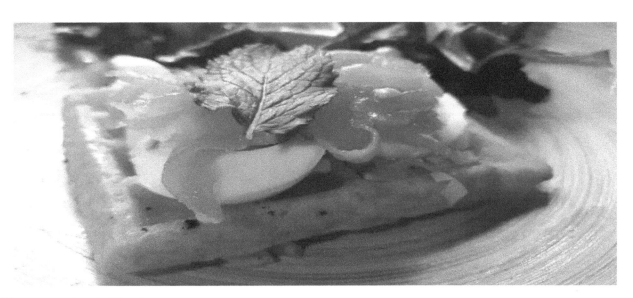

Time required: 10 min

Portions provided: 3

Ingredients:

- 300 g grated potato
- 1 egg yolk
- 20 ml milk
- 199 g corn flour
- 2 tablespoons oil
- 40 g parmesan cheese
- 2 packet smoked salmon
- Salt to your liking

Preparation:

1. Spread oil or butter on the waffle maker so it doesn't stick and start making waffles. Let the waffle maker heat up between waffles and oil it if it starts to dry.

2. The potato should be washed, peeled, and grated.

3. Wring it out thoroughly and dry it with a clean rag.

4. Mix the egg yolk with the milk in a mixing bowl, then add the cornmeal, grated cheese, and a tablespoon of oil when it's finished.

5. While the waffle maker is heating, apply the grated potato to the previous mixture and stir well.

6. Serve the waffles with smoked salmon and your favorite sauce, or put the salmon, hard-boiled egg, capers, chopped onion, and greek yogurt with dill on top.

7. Note: based on how liquid the dough is, you can need to adjust the flour, so I suggest gradually adding the milk and flour.

FRIED PICKLE CHAFFLE STICKS

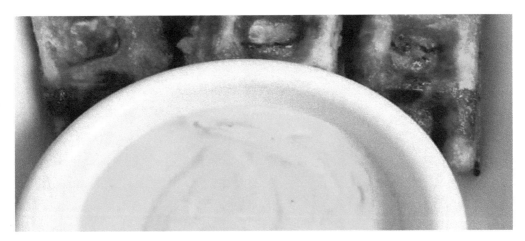

Time required: 5 min

Portions provided: 1

Ingredients:

- 1 egg, large

- 1/4 cup pork panko

- 1/2 cup mozzarella

- 1 tablespoon pickle juice

- 6-8 thin pickle slices

Preparation:

1. Combine all of the ingredients.

2. Spread a thin layer of batter on the waffle iron.

3. Remove excess pickle juice with a paper towel.

4. Add pickle slices and a thin layer of mix on top.

5. Cook for 4 minutes.

6. Ranch dressing with Frank's hot sauce as a dipping sauce

Nutrition Facts: Calories 465; Carbohydrates 3.3g; Fiber 1.4g; Sugar 1.5g; Fat 22.7g; Protein 59.2g

DAIRY-FREE WHOLE WHEAT WAFFLES

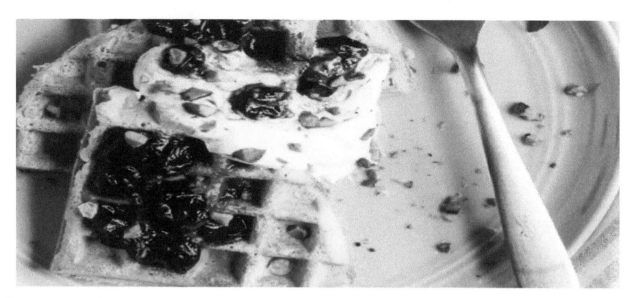

Time required: 40 min

Portions provided: 4

Ingredients:

- 1 cup all-purpose flour
- 1/2 cup whole wheat flour
- 2 teaspoons baking powder
- 1/2 teaspoon ground cinnamon
- 1/4 teaspoon ground allspice
- 1/2 teaspoon kosher salt
- 1 large egg
- 1/4 cup coconut oil, melted and slightly cooled
- 1 1/4 cups unsweetened almond milk beverage
- 1 teaspoon vanilla extract
- 2 tablespoons maple syrup

Preparation:

1. Pre - heat a waffle iron to high temperature. Mix the all-purpose flour, whole wheat flour, baking powder, cinnamon, allspice, and kosher salt together in a medium mixing bowl until well mixed. Whisk the egg in a separate dish. Then add the melted coconut oil, almond milk, vanilla extract, and maple syrup and mix to combine. Mix the wet and dry ingredients together gently until just combined; do not overmix.

2. Immediately pour 12 cup batter into the waffle iron's center and spread it out to within 12 inch of the sides; cook according to the waffle iron's directions.

3. Remove the cooked waffles from the pan and put them on a baking sheet in a single layer. Waffles can be made to order, or cooked waffles can be kept warm in a 300°f oven. Serve with the toppings of your choice.

NORWEGIAN WAFFLE

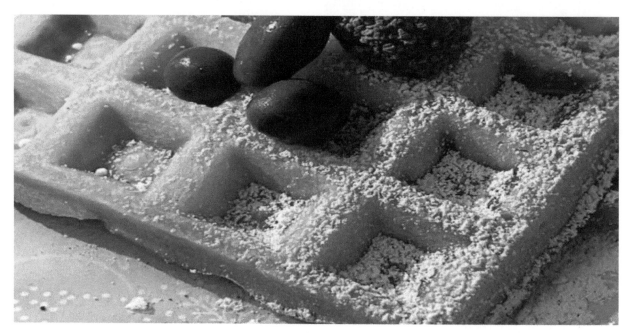

Time required: 15 min

Portions provided: 1

Ingredients:

- 250 gr all-purpose flour
- 1 egg
- 1 tsp sour cream
- 1/4 tbsp baking powder
- 1/2 tsp vanilla
- 1 tbsp sugar
- 1 cup fresh milk
- 75-100 gr butter (melted)
- Salt
- Water to dissolve
- Butter to grease waffle maker

Preparation:

1. In a mixing bowl, whisk together the eggs, bp, vanilla, and sugar. Mix on high until foamy, then slowly drizzle in the sour cream and milk.

2. Gradually add the flour. Slowly pour in the water until it reaches a decent consistency, then add the butter (keep mixing).

3. Using butter, grease the waffle maker (even though it's a nonstick pan!). Prepare your waffle.

SALTY HAM AND CHEESE WAFFLES

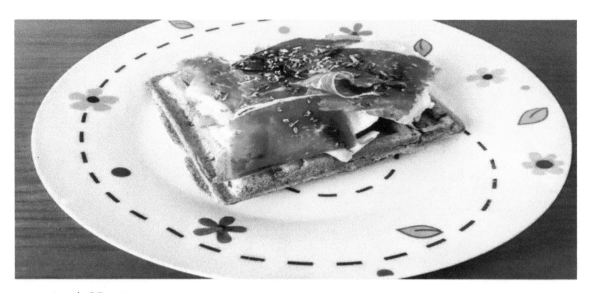

Time required: 25 min

Portions provided: 4-5

Ingredients:

- 240 gr wholemeal flour
- 400 ml fresh milk (or whatever you have)
- 3 eggs
- 2 teaspoons royal type yeast
- 1 tablespoon extra virgin olive oil

Toppings

- 3-4 balls mozzarella cheese
- 1 package sliced Serrano ham
- To taste oregano

Preparation:

1. In a mixing bowl, combine all of the dough's ingredients.

2. Mix them together until you have a smooth, lump-free dough. It's possible to make it with a robot, a blender, a blender... All performs admirably.

3. When the waffle iron is hot, pour a couple of tablespoons of batter into each of the holes. Close it and wait until they're finished, then serve them on a plate, repeating the process with the rest of the dough until it's gone.

4. Insert half a ball of sliced mozzarella, serrano ham, and oregano to taste on top of each waffle.

SALTY SALMON AND MOZZARELLA WAFFLES

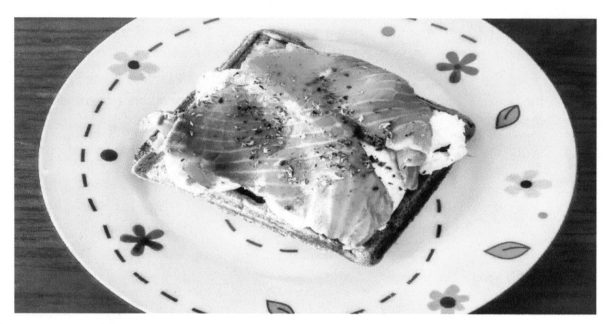

Time required: 25 min

Portions provided: 8

Ingredients:

- 240 gr wholemeal flour

- 400 ml fresh milk (or whatever you have)

- 3 eggs

- 2 teaspoons royal type yeast

- 1 tablespoon extra virgin olive oil

- Toppings

- 3-4 balls mozzarella cheese

- Slices smoked salmon

- To taste dried dill (optional but highly recommended)

Preparation:

1. Place all of the dough's ingredients in a jar that can be beaten.

2. Mix until a smooth, lump-free dough is formed. You may use a drone, a mixer, a blender... It looks great with everything.

3. When the waffle iron is hot, fill each hole with a couple of tablespoons of batter. Close it and leave them there until they're finished, then serve them on a plate, repeating the process with the rest of the dough until it's gone.

4. Place half a ball of sliced mozzarella, smoked salmon, and dried dill to taste on top of each waffle.

CINNAMON ROLL CHAFFLE

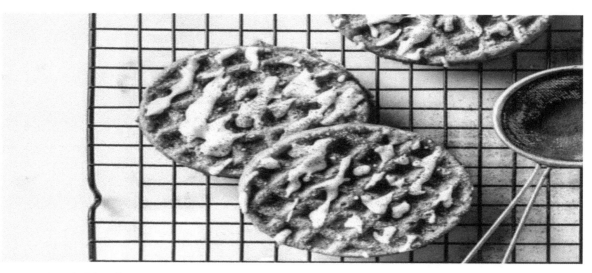

Time required: 30 min

Portions provided: 4

Ingredients:

- ½ cup (56g) shredded mozzarella cheese
- 2 tbsp (24g) golden monk fruit sweetener
- 2 tbsp (32g) No-Sugar-Added SunButter
- 1 egg
- 1 tbsp (7g) coconut flour
- 2 tsp cinnamon
- ¼ tsp vanilla extract
- ⅛ tsp baking powder

For the frosting:

- ¼ cup (48g) powdered monk fruit sweetener
- 1 tbsp (0.5 oz) cream cheese
- ¾ tbsp (~11g) butter, melted
- ¼ tsp vanilla extract or ⅛ tsp maple extract
- 1 tbsp (15 mL) unsweetened coconut milk (from a container)

For the coating:

- 1 tsp cinnamon
- 1 tsp (4g) golden monk fruit sweetener

Preparation:

1. Preheat the waffle iron as you prepare the batter and frosting.

2. Batter: Combine all batter ingredients in a big mixing bowl. Enable 3-5 minutes for the batter to set in the tub.

3. To make the frosting, whisk together powdered monk fruit sweetener, cream cheese, butter, and vanilla or maple extract in a separate small mixing bowl until smooth. Pour in the coconut milk and whisk all together again until everything is well mixed. Remove from the equation.

4. Finish by spraying a preheated waffle iron liberally with nonstick cooking spray. Divide the chaffle batter into three portions and spoon one into the waffle iron, leaving a slight gap around the edge since the batter can expand during cooking. Cook for 2-4 minutes, or until chaffle is golden brown.

5. Enable 30 seconds for the chaffle to cool in the waffle iron before carefully removing the chaffle from the waffle iron with a fork and transferring to a plate. Sprinkle chaffles with cinnamon and monk fruit sweetener coating while still wet. Drizzle icing over chaffles until they've cooled slightly.

Notes:

1. If you don't have a nut allergy, unsweetened almond butter or unsweetened peanut butter can be used in place of SunButter in a 1:1 ratio.

2. Refrigerate the keto chaffles in an airtight jar or freezer bag for up to 3 days before eating.

3. To keep these chaffles from sticking together in the freezer, place them in a freezer bag or an airtight container and separate them with parchment paper. Keep for up to 2 months in the freezer.

4. Reheating refrigerated or frozen chaffles: To heat it up refrigerated chaffles, put them in a toaster (only use a toaster if you haven't pre-drizzled the chaffles with icing), a preheated toaster oven, or a preheated oven and heat until thoroughly warmed. I wouldn't recommend reheating them in the microwave because they will become very chewy. If using frozen chaffles, thaw them in the refrigerator before reheating.

KETO PEANUT BUTTER CUP CHAFFLE

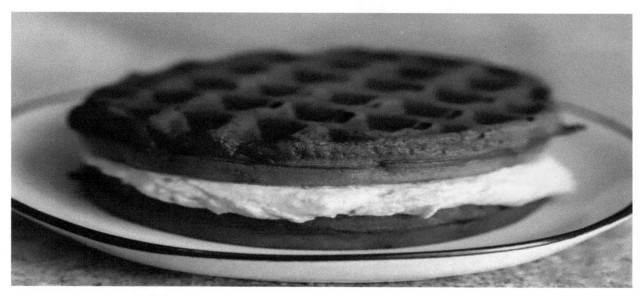

Time required: 6 min

Portions provided: 1 serving

Ingredients:

- 1 Egg
- 1 tbsp Heavy Cream
- 1 tbsp Unsweetened Cocoa
- 1 tbsp Lakanto Powdered Sweetener
- 1 tsp Coconut Flour
- 1/2 tsp Vanilla Extract
- 1/2 tsp Cake Batter Flavor (we use this)
- 1/4 tsp Baking Powder
- Peanut Butter Filling
- 3 tbsp All natural Peanut Butter
- 2 tsp Lakanto Powdered Sweetener
- 2 tbsp Heavy Cream

Preparation:

1. Preheat the mini waffle iron.
2. Combine all chaffle ingredients in a small mixing bowl.
3. Pour half of the chaffle batter into the waffle iron's middle. Allow for 3-5 minutes of cooking time.
4. Remove carefully and repeat for the second chaffle. Allow for a few minutes for the chaffles to crisp up.
5. To make the peanut butter filling, whisk together all of the ingredients and distribute evenly between the chaffles.

Nutrition Facts: *Per Serving:* Calories 264; Carbohydtrates 7.25g; Net Carbohydrates 4.5g; Fat 21.6g; Fiber 2.75g; Protein 9.45g

SNACKS APPETIZER RECIPES

KETO OREO CHAFFLES

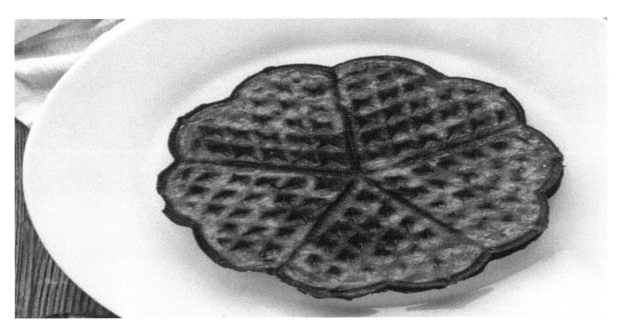

Time required: 15 min

Portions provided: 2

Ingredients:

- 1/2 cup Sugar-Free Chocolate Chips
- 1/2 cup Butter
- 3 Eggs
- 1/4 cup Truvia, or other sweetener
- 1 teaspoon Vanilla extract
- Cream Cheese Frosting
- 4 ounces Butter, room temperature
- 4 ounces Cream Cheese, room temperature
- 1/2 cup Powdered Swerve
- 1/4 cup Heavy Whipping Cream
- 1 teaspoon Vanilla extract

Preparation:

1. Melt butter and chocolate in a microwave-safe bowl for around 1 minute. Remove the lid and give it a good stir. The heat from the butter and chocolate can be used to melt the remaining clumps. You've overcooked the chocolate if you microwave it until it's fully melted. So grab a spoon and get to work. If necessary, add another 10 seconds, but stir thoroughly first.

2. In a mixing bowl, whisk together the eggs, sweetener, and vanilla extract until light and fluffy.

3. In a slow stream, pour the melted butter and chocolate into the mixing bowl and beat until well combined.

4. In a Dash Mini waffle iron, cook for 7-8 minutes, or until crispy, with around 1/4 of the mixture.

5. While they're cooking, make the frosting.

6. In the bowl of a food processor, combine all of the frosting ingredients and process until smooth and fluffy. To achieve the desired consistency, you may need to add a little more cream.

7. To make your Oreo chaffle, generously pipe or spread the frosting in between two chaffles.

8. Two full-size Oreo chaffles or four mini Oreo chaffles should be enough.

9. Make sure the waffle maker isn't overflowing! It will result in a colossal mess and the waste of batter. In a Dash Mini, use no more than 1/4 cup batter.

10. Allow for some cooling time before eating and frosting the waffles. They will crisp up as a result of this.

11. Create your frosting with room temperature cream cheese and butter.

Nutrition Facts: Calories 1381; Carbohydrates 14g; Protein 17g; Fat 146g; Fiber 5g; Sugar 3g

WAFFLE BREAD

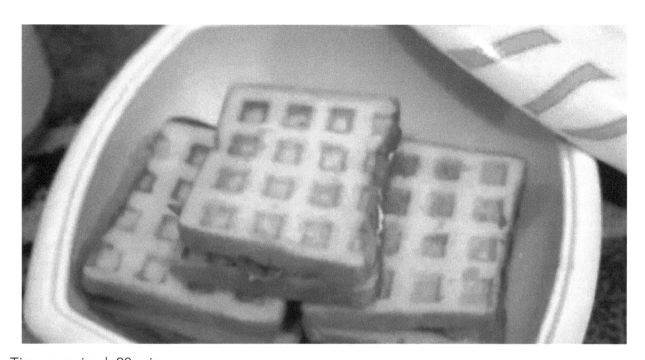

Time required: 20 min

Portions provided: 4

Ingredients:

- Slice of bread
- Mince
- Cucumber
- Bama
- Onion
- Spice
- Spice
- Scott hood
- Butter
- Waffle maker
- Mayonnaise

Preparation:

1. Place the bread on a waffle iron and spread the butter on it.

2. Place the minced meat in a frying pan with the seasonings, spices, and a little oil, cover, and set aside.

3. Slice the onion, add a little water and oil, the spices, and the onion, and set aside.

4. Cucumber should be cut, and meat should be mixed with mayonnaise.

5. Place the cucumber on one piece of bread, then the heart, then the onion, and top with another waffle of bread.

THE WAFFLE-BURGER

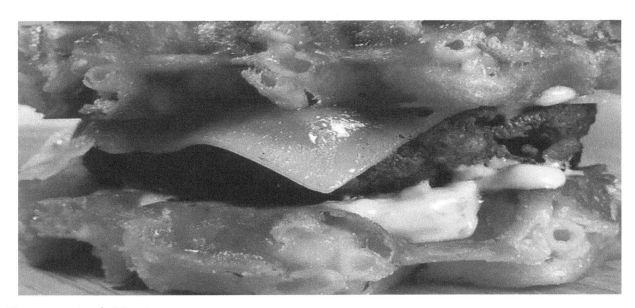

Time required: 10 min

Portions provided: 1

Ingredients:

- 2 waffles
- 1 beef burger
- 1 slice cheese
- Fried onion
- Honey
- Mustard

Preparation:

1. Toast the waffles with honey on top.
2. Cook the hamburger and top it with cheese, mustard, and fried onions.
3. Finally, we put the waffle-hamburger together.

SQUARE CHEESEBURGER WAFFLES

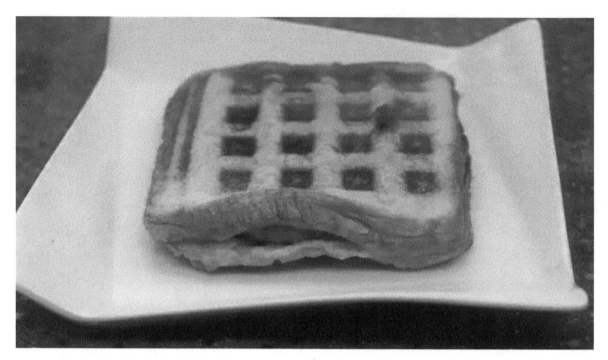

Time required: 30 min

Portions provided: 2

Ingredients:

- 4 slices bread
- 2 meat burgers (or whatever you like)
- 4 slices of cheese
- 1 tomato
- Olive oil
- Salt

Preparation:

1. While hamburgers can be cooked in a frying pan, we prefer to use a waffle iron.

2. To prevent staining the waffle iron, we lined it with baking paper and crushed the hamburger a little to make it square and fit it to the size of the bread.

3. Season both burgers and cook them in a waffle iron for 10-15 minutes, with baking paper underneath and on top (you can spray the paper with a little oil).

4. As my normal tomato sauce is being prepared.

5. You wash and cut a ripe tomato, season with salt and olive oil, and crush and spread sliced bread on one side of the bread. On two of the tomato-smeared ears, we put a slice of cheese.

6. When the hamburgers are finished, we put both of them on the cheese-filled slices and cover them with the two remaining slices.

7. The remaining two slices of bread are used to coat the slices.

8. You put it in the waffle iron for about 10 minutes, or until the toasting point is to our liking.

9. Due to the thickness of our waffles, the waffle iron will be a little open, so you can place a weight on top or tie the waffle iron with a string to help it close more tightly.

10. Heat the dish before serving.

HOT DOG WAFFLES

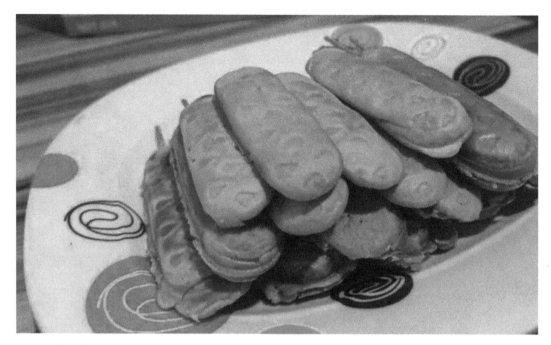

Time required: 20 min

Portions provided: 2

Ingredients:

- 2 cups of flour
- 2 tablespoons of sugar
- 1 teaspoon of salt
- 4 teaspoons of baking powder
- 3 tablespoons of butter
- 1 large egg
- 4-6 sausages
- 1 1/2 cup of warm milk
- Flavor of vanilla

Preparation:

1. In a mixing bowl, combine the flour, sugar, salt, and baking powder.

2. Mix the milk powder with warm water, then apply a teaspoon of flavoring to the egg mixer.

3. Combine the wet and dry ingredients in a blender until smooth. Remove the sausages from the casings and cut them in half.

4. Place the skewers on the waffle iron and preheat it when it is hot. Fill it with the batter. In the middle, position the sausage and cook until golden brown and cooked through.

HOT DOG WAFFLES CHOCOLATE

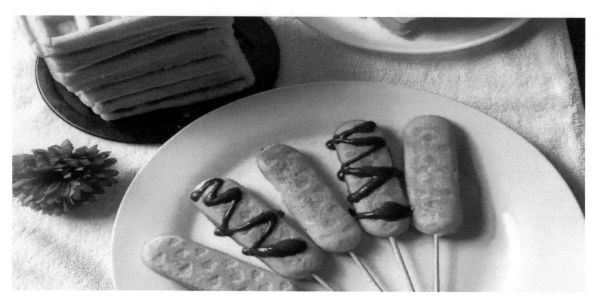

Time required: 20 min

Portions provided: 3

Ingredients:

- 2 cups of flour
- 3/4 cup of sugar
- 90 g of margarine
- 4 teaspoons of baking powder
- 11/2 cup of milk
- 2 large eggs
- Bamboo skewers
- Chocolate sauce
- Gold coins to decorate

Preparation:

1. Combine all of your dry ingredients in a large mixing bowl.

2. In a microwave or on the burner, melt the margarine.

3. Toss the dry ingredients with the melted butter, milk, and vanilla extract.

4. Use a hand mixer or a whisk to combine the ingredients. It is not necessary for the dough to be smooth.

5. Fill each hole in half with batter and cook until the red light appears in your hot dog machine, stacking bamboo skewers if desired.

6. Serve with chocolate sauce or simple.

KETO CHAFFLE BLT SANDWICH

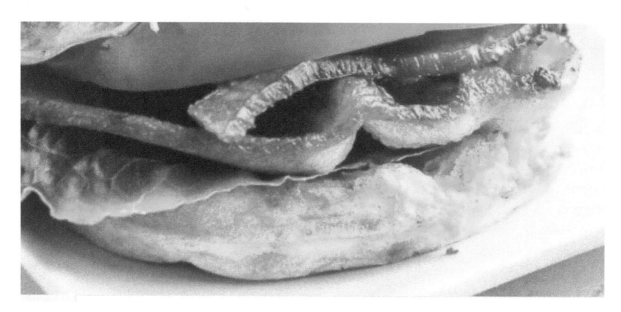

Time required: 13 min

Portions provided: 2

Ingredients:

- 1 egg
- 1/2 cup Cheddar cheese, shredded
- For the sandwich
- 2 strips bacon
- 1-2 slices tomato
- 2-3 pieces lettuce
- 1 tablespoon mayonnaise

Preparation:

1. Pre - heat the waffle maker as directed by the manufacturer.

2. Combine the egg and shredded cheese in a shallow mixing bowl. Stir until it is well blended.

3. Half of the waffle batter should be poured into the waffle maker. Cook until golden brown, around 3-4 minutes. Continue with the other half of the batter.

4. Cook the bacon in a large skillet over medium heat until crispy, turning as needed. Remove to a plate lined with paper towels to drain.

5. Assemble the sandwich by layering lettuce, tomato, and mayonnaise between two slices of bread. Have fun!

Nutrition Facts: *Per Serving:* Calories 238; Carbohydrates 2g; Total Fat 18g; Saturated Fat 9g; Trans Fat 0g; Unsaturated Fat 7g; Cholesterol 143mg; Sodium 554mg; Fiber 0g; Sugar 1g; Protein 17g

Notes: You may be able to cook the whole batch of batter in one waffle if you use a larger waffle maker. The size of your computer will determine this.

MIXED SANDWICH WITH SALTY POTATO AND ZUCCHINI WAFFLE

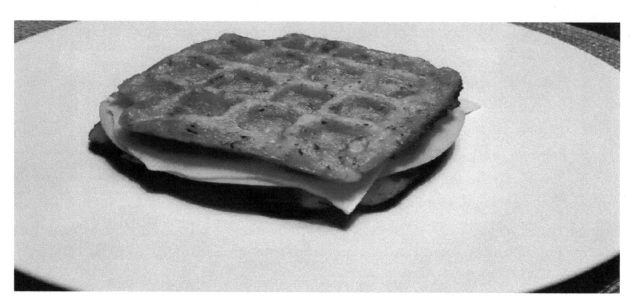

Time required: 20 min

Portions provided: 2

Ingredients:

- Cheese
- 1 large potato
- 1/2 zucchini
- 3 tablespoons flour
- 1 tablespoon oil
- 1 teaspoon baking powder
- 1 teaspoon garlic powder
- 1 pinch salt
- York ham

Preparation:

1. Microwave the potato in a covered jar for 7 minutes after peeling and chopping it into small squares.
2. Grate the zucchini, toss it in with the potato, and cook for another 5 minutes in the microwave.
3. Using a fork, mash all together.
4. Knead in the remaining ingredients, except the filling (ham and cheese), until a dough forms that does not stick to your hands.
5. Allow a portion of dough to brown in each hole of the waffle iron.
6. Fill with ham and cheese or whatever other toppings we choose.

KETO CHAFFLE (CHEESE WAFFLE) PLUS OMAD SANDWICH

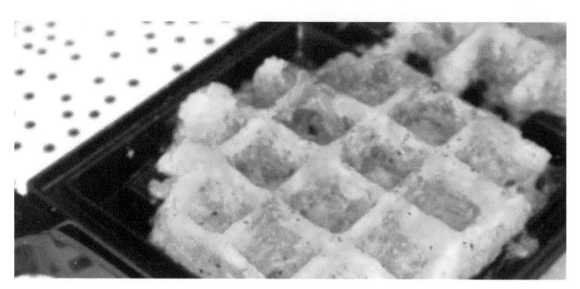

Time required: 10 min

Portions provided: 2

Ingredients:

For the waffle:

- 3/4 cup (75g) shredded cheese (of your choice)
- 1 medium egg
- 1 tsp psyllium husk
- salt/pepper
- hot sauce (optional)

For the sandwich:

- 4 slices bacon
- 4 slices ham
- 4 slices prosciutto
- 5-6 slices salami
- 5-6 slices pepperoni
- mustard
- mayonnaise

Preparation:

1. In a bowl, whisk together the egg, cheese, salt, pepper, psyllium husk and optional hot sauce.

2. Bring your waffle maker to temperature before pouring the batter evenly into the waffle maker.

3. Cook for 2-3 minutes, or longer depending on how crispy you want it

4. Take out and enjoy as is or top with the sandwich ingredients for a filling, fat filled meal!

PIZZA WAFFLES

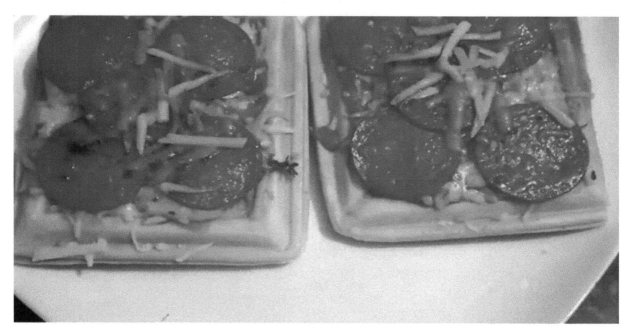

Time required: 40 min

Portions provided: 4

Ingredients:

- Waffle batter
- 270 gm flour
- 125 ml milk
- 75 gm butter at room temperature
- 1/2 beaten egg
- 4 gm dry yeast
- 6 gm salt
- Stuffed
- Fried tomato
- 4 cheeses
- Pepperoni and oregano

Preparation:

1. Heat the milk and cut it in half in a tub. Combine half of the milk, yeast, and a tablespoon of flour in a mixing bowl. Stir well and set aside for 15 minutes.

2. Place the flour in a cup, make a hole in the middle, and add the salt, egg, and yeast around it. Knead thoroughly.

3. Remove the butter from the bowl and stir well. Knead until an elastic dough forms, then set aside to rest for at least an hour.

4. Remove it from the bowl and split it into four equal bits.

5. When the waffle iron is ready, form the portions of the waffle iron's shape and bake them.

6. Put the tomato sauce, oregano, cheese, pepperoni, and a little cheese in the filling. Place in a preheated oven at 150°f and bake until the cheese is melted.

KRISPY KREME COPYCAT CHAFFLE RECIPE (GLAZED RASPBERRY JELLY FILLED DONUT)

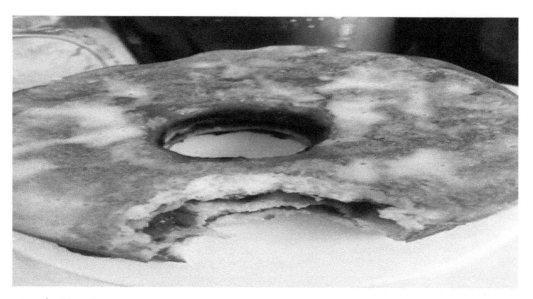

Time required: 49 min

Portions provided: 2

Ingredients:

KRISPY KREME COPYCAT CHAFFLE

- 1 egg

- 1/4 cup mozzarella cheese, shredded

- 2 T cream cheese, softened

- 1 T sweetener

- 1 T almond flour

- 1/2 tsp Baking Powder

- 20 drops glazed donut flavoring by OOOFlavors

- Raspberry Jelly Filling Ingredients

- 1/4 cup raspberries

- 1 tsp chia seeds

- 1 tsp confectioners sweetener

- Donut Glaze Ingredients

- 1 tsp powdered sweetener

- A few drops of water or heavy whipping cream

CAP'N CRUNCH CEREAL CHAFFLE CAKE

- 1 egg
- 2 tablespoons almond flour
- 1/2 teaspoon coconut flour
- 1 tablespoon butter, melted
- 1 tablespoon cream cheese, room temp
- 20 drops Captain Cereal flavoring
- 1/4 teaspoon vanilla extract
- 1/4 teaspoon baking powder
- 1 tablespoon confectioners sweetener
- 1/8 teaspoon xanthan gum
- Keto Greek Chicken Bowl Recipe

Preparation:

1. Preheat the waffle maker for mini waffles.

2. Combine all of the ingredients in a blender or food processor and process until smooth and fluffy. Allow for a few minutes of resting time for the flour to absorb the moisture.

3. Cook for around 2 1/2 minutes with 2 to 3 tablespoons of batter in your waffle maker.

4. Top with new whipped cream and syrup (to which I added 10 drops of Captain cereal flavoring)!

Nutrition Facts: Calories 154; Total Carbohydrates 5.6g; Net Carbohydrates 4g; Fiber 1.6g; Sugar 2.7g; Fat 11.2g; Protein 4.6g

HAWAIIAN WAFFLE PIZZA / PIZZA FLIP

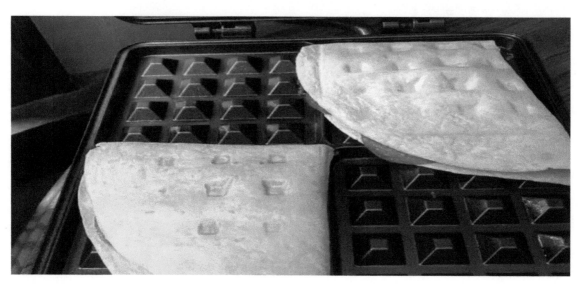

Time required: 10 min

Portions provided: 2-3

Ingredients:

- 1 large soft tortilla
- Try the pizza sauce
- Taste the peppers
- To taste canadian bacon
- Drain the pineapple chunks
- Try the mozzarella

Preparation:

1. Waffle iron should be preheated.
2. Cook until the cheese has melted and the mixture is thoroughly cooked. Remember to spray the waffle iron with a nun's wand after each use.

KETO PIZZA CHAFFLE

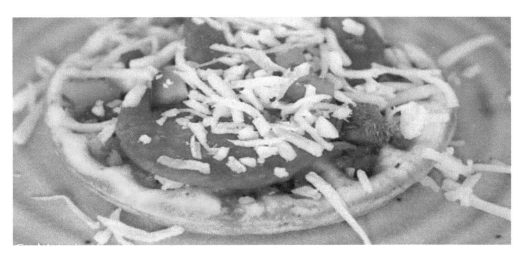

Time required: 30 min

Portions provided: 2

Ingredients:

- 1 egg
- 1/2 cup mozzarella cheese shredded
- Just a pinch of Italian seasoning
- No sugar added pizza sauce about 1 tablespoon
- Top with more shredded cheese pepperoni (or any of your favorite toppings)

Preparation:

1. Preheat the Dash waffle maker.

2. In a small bowl, whip the egg and seasonings together.

3. Mix in the shredded cheese.

4. Add a tsp of shredded cheese to the preheated waffle maker and let it cook for about 30 seconds. This will help to create a more crisp crust.

5. Add half the mixture to the waffle maker and cook it for about 4 minutes until it's golden brown and slightly crispy!

6. Remove the waffle and add the remaining mixture to the waffle maker to make the second chaffle.

7. Pre - heat the waffle maker Dash.

8. Whisk together the egg and seasonings in a small bowl.

9. Add the shredded cheese and stir to combine.

10. Cook for about 30 seconds with a tsp of shredded cheese in a preheated waffle maker. This will aid in the creation of a crispier crust.

11. Half of the mixture should be added to the waffle maker and cooked for 4 minutes, or until golden brown and slightly crispy!

12. Pull the waffle from the waffle maker and apply the remaining mixture to create the second chaffle.

13. Add a tablespoon of pizza sauce, shredded cheese, and pepperoni to the top of the pizza. Microwave it for about 20 seconds on high, and voila!

Nutrition Facts: *Per Serving:* Calories 76; Carbohydrates 4.1g; Fat 4,3g; Protein 5.5g; Fiber 1.2g; Sugar 1.9g

POULTRY RECIPES

BUFFALO CHICKEN CHAFFLE RECIPE FOR LOW CARB WAFFLES

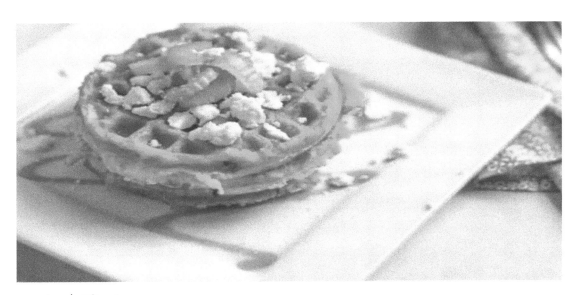

Time required: 19 min

Portions provided: 2

Ingredients:

- ¼ cup almond flour
- 1 teaspoon baking powder
- 2 large eggs
- ½ cup chicken, shredded
- ¼ cup mozzarella cheese, shredded
- ¼ cup Frank's Red Hot Sauce + optional 1 tablespoon for topping
- ¾ cup sharp cheddar cheese, shredded
- ¼ cup feta cheese, crumbled
- ¼ cup celery, diced

Preparation:

1. Whisk the baking powder into the almond flour in a small mixing bowl and set aside.
2. Preheat waffle iron to medium/high heat and liberally coat with low-carb non-stick spray.
3. Add eggs to a big mixing bowl and whisk until frothy.
4. To begin, beat in the hot sauce until well combined.
5. Combine flour and eggs in a mixing bowl and stir until just mixed.
6. Finally, stir in the shredded cheeses until thoroughly mixed.
7. In a large mixing bowl, combine the shredded chicken and the mayonnaise.
8. Cook chaffle batter until it browns on the outside in a preheated waffle maker. It takes about 4 minutes.
9. Pull the waffle maker from the oven and repeat Step 7 until all of the batter has been used.
10. Serve chaffles with feta cheese, celery, and/or hot sauce on top.

Nutrition Facts: *Per Serving:* Calories 675; Carbohydrates 8g; Total Fat 52g; Satured Fat 24g; Trans Fat 1g; Unsatured Fat 22g; Cholesterol 330mg; Fiber 2g; Sugar 3g; Protein 44g

ERIC'S CHICKEN AND WAFFLES WITH BOURBON MAPLE SYRUP

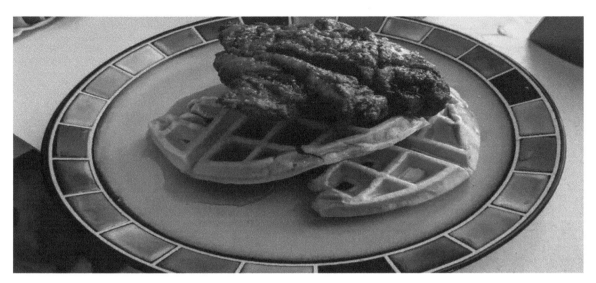

Time required: 1 hour and 40 minutes

Portions provided: 3-4

Ingredients:

- 6 chicken thighs
- liters of buttermilk
- 2 tablespoons sriracha
- For the oil
- Peanut oil
- A few sprigs of fresh rosemary
- Some fresh sage
- Some fresh thyme
- 1 small garlic clove
- To dredge
- 3 cups all-purpose flour
- 2/3 cup cornstarch
- 1 teaspoon baking powder
- 1 tablespoon of salt

- 2 tablespoons of paprika
- 2 tablespoons onion powder
- 2 tablespoons garlic powder
- 1 teaspoon dried oregano
- 1 teaspoon dried basil
- 1 teaspoon of white pepper
- 2 teaspoons cayenne pepper
- 4 teaspoons light brown sugar
- For the bourbon maple syrup
- 2 ounces bourbon
- 8 ounces maple syrup
- 3 tablespoons of butter
- For the waffles
- 2 cups whole milk
- 2 1/2 cups all-purpose flour
- 1 tablespoon baking powder
- 3 spoonfuls of sugar
- 1/2 teaspoon cinnamon
- 2 eggs, whites, and yolks separately
- 1/2 cup vegetable oil
- 1 teaspoon vanilla extract

Preparation:

For the chicken:

1. In a big mixing bowl, combine 1 liter buttermilk and sriracha. Turn the chicken parts to coat them in the sauce. Refrigerate for at least 4 hours after covering. I tend to prepare them the night before and leave them to rest overnight.

2. In a big mixing bowl, combine all of the ingredients for the excavator, season with salt and pepper, and divide into two containers. Before frying, you'll make a dry and a wet excavator. Place the remaining half liter of buttermilk in a box as well.

3. Remove the chicken from the freezer, remove the chunks from the buttermilk mixture, and drain any excess liquid in a colander.

4. Each piece of chicken should be dragged to a bowl of flour, blotted dry, dipped in fresh buttermilk, drained, and then dragged to a second bowl of flour. Take out the frill and set it aside.

5. The amount of oil you use will be determined by the size of the frying pan you use. I use a big pot for spaghetti and pour a few inches of fat into it, making sure to sit underneath and halfway fill it. Turn the flame to a medium setting and add the oil additives to raise the temperature to 350-360 degrees. When the oil is heated, the herbs and garlic give it a taste.

6. One by one, add the chicken bits. Overcrowding the pot may cause the temperature to drop. Cook for about 20 minutes, turning the chicken parts every few minutes, until golden brown. Rest the finished chicken for 10 minutes on a rack to drip.

7. To make the syrup: in a small saucepan, combine the bourbon and maple syrup and cook over high heat to extract the alcohol. It should take about 5 minutes to complete this task. Remove the pan from the heat and stir in the butter until thoroughly combined. Set aside, whether it's hot or cold.

For waffles:

1. In a mixing bowl, combine the flour, baking powder, sugar, salt, and cinnamon.

2. Separate the egg whites and beat them until firm in a separate tub.

3. In a separate cup, whisk together the egg yolks, vegetable oil, milk, and vanilla extract, then combine with the flour mixture.

4. Combine the egg whites, yolks, and flour mixture in a mixing bowl. Cook them on the waffle iron of your choosing once they've been mixed.

DESSERT RECIPES

CHOCOLATE KETO CHAFFLES

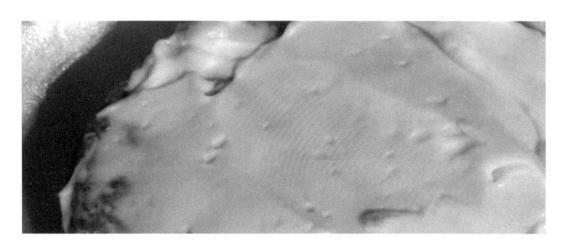

Time required: 10 min

Portions provided: 2

Ingredients:

- 4 oz. of Cream Cheese.
- 4 of Eggs.
- e 2 tsp of Vanilla.
- 2 Tbs of Swerve sugar Substitute.
- 4 Tbs of Rice Flour.
- It's 1 1/2 tsp of Baking powder.
- 1 Tbs of 100 % Cocoa Powder.
- Pinch of Salt.

For the topping:

- 4 oz of Cream Cheese.
- 1/4 Stick of butter (Room Temperature).
- 1 Tbs of Swerve (sugar Substitute).

Preparation:

1. In a waffle maker, preheat 4 waffles.
2. Mix all chaffle ingredients in a blender or in a mixing bowl until well combined.
3. Brush the waffle maker with melted butter or spray it with olive oil.
4. Pour enough chaffle batter into the waffle maker to cover the rim. (Your experience will tell you how much.)
5. Four minutes in the oven, or a little longer if you like crispier chaffles.
6. Place on a cooling rack to cool.
7. To make the topping, combine all of the ingredients and spread on cooled chaffles.
8. Chaffles can be frozen and reheated at a later time.

Notes: Keto chocolate chips are used in these Chocolate Chip chaffles. White, milk, or dark chips may be used. Whichever one you want! Don't forget to drizzle some of our sugar-free syrup on top of your chaffles. Right now, keto chaffle recipes are all over the place, and they're not going anywhere anytime soon. This is due to the fact that chaffles are both simple to make and flexible.

LOW-CARB CHOCOLATE CHIP VANILLA CHAFFLES

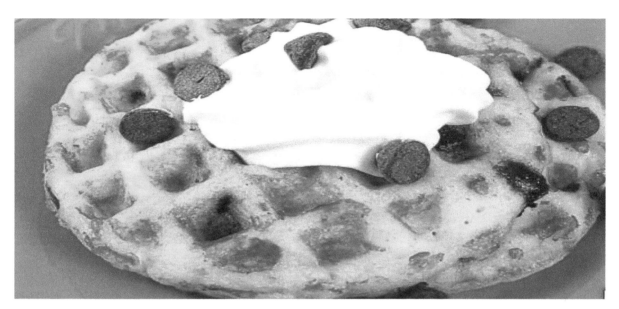

Time required: 5 minutes

Portions provided: 1

Ingredients:

- 1/2 cup pre-shredded/grated mozzarella
- 1 eggs - medium
- 1 tbsp granulated sweetener of choice or more to your taste
- 1 tsp vanilla extract
- 2 tbsp almond meal/flour
- 1 tbsp sugar-free chocolate chips or cacao nibs

Preparation:

1. In a mixing bowl, combine all of the ingredients.
2. Preheat the waffle maker for mini waffles. When the waffle maker is wet, spray it with olive oil and pour half of the batter into it. Cook for 2-4 minutes before removing and repeating the process. Per recipe, you should be able to make 2 mini-chaffles.
3. Garnish, serve, and savor.

EASY DOUBLE CHOCOLATE CHAFFLES

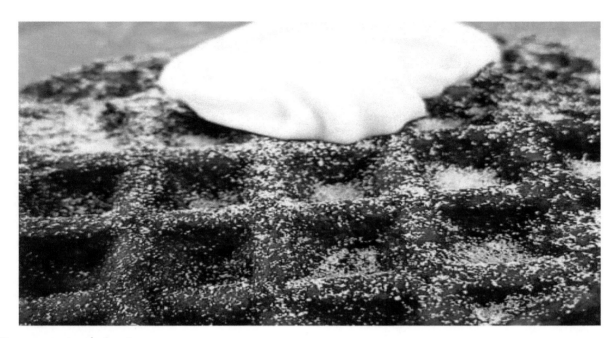

Time required: 4 min

Portions provided: 1

Ingredients:

- Double Chocolate Chaffles
- 1 eggs - medium
- 1/2 cup pre-shredded/grated mozzarella
- 1 tbsp granulated sweetener of choice or more to your taste
- 1 tsp vanilla
- 2 tbsp almond meal/flour
- 1 tbsp sugar-free chocolate chips or cacao nibs
- 2 tbsp cocoa powder unsweetened
- 1 tsp heavy/double cream

Preparation:

1. In a mixing bowl, combine the ingredients for your preferred flavor.

2. Preheat the waffle iron. Spray the mini-waffle maker with olive oil once it's hot, and pour half the batter into it (or the entire batter into a large waffle maker).

3. Cook for 2-4 minutes before removing and repeating the process. Per recipe, you should be able to make 2 mini-chaffles or 1 big chaffle.

4. Garnish, serve, and savor.

Nutrition Facts: *Per Serving:* Calories 337.7;   Carbohydrates 11.2g 4%; Fat 23.3g 36%; Sodium 416.6mg 18%; Potassium 270.6mg 8%; Fiber 4.8g 20%; Sugar 2g 2%; Protein 24.3g 49%

FIT CHOCOLATE WAFFLE WITH NOUGAT ICE CREAM 2 INGREDIENTS

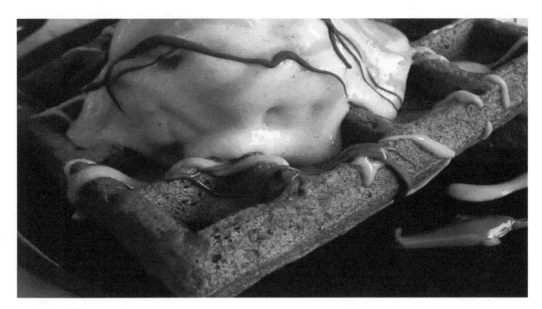

Time required: 10 minutes

Portions provided: 1

Ingredients:

- 1 egg
- 1 tbsp (35g) yogurt or whipped cheese
- 1 tsp (10 g) agave syrup (or other sweetener)
- 20 g oatmeal
- 10 g almond flour (or more oats)
- 10 g pure cocoa powder
- 1/2 tsp baking powder
- Frozen
- 1 frozen banana (100g)
- 20 g almond cream
- 1 pinch cinnamon

Preparation:

1. Thoroughly combine all of the waffle ingredients and cook them in a preheated waffle maker greased with a little coconut oil or butter.

2. For the ice cream, we simply smash the ingredients until they are fully homogeneous.

3. The waffles are served with ice cream, almond cream, and melted chocolate, and that's it!

HEALTHY WAFFLES WITH CHOCOLATE SYRUP

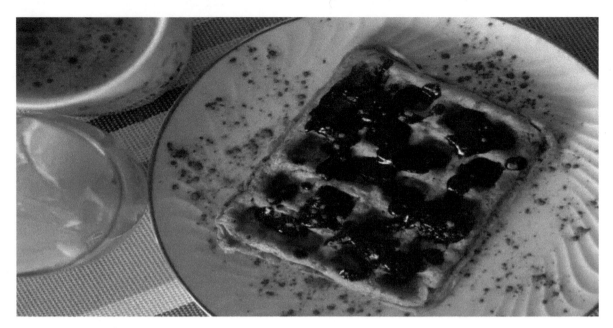

Time required: 10 minutes

Portions provided: 1

Ingredients:

- 30 gr flour
- 2 egg whites
- 2 tablespoons quark cheese
- 1 dessert spoon of cinnamon
- Vanilla scent
- 1 c / s agave syrup

Preparation:

1. In a blender glass, combine all of the ingredients and beat until a thick, lump-free mixture forms.

2. 1 teaspoon defatted cocoa powder, 3 tablespoons sugar, a drop of agave syrup to sweeten, and a pinch of corn flour to thicken the syrup reduce the heat to low and continue to mix until the sauce thickens.

LOW CARB GLAZED DONUT CHAFFLE

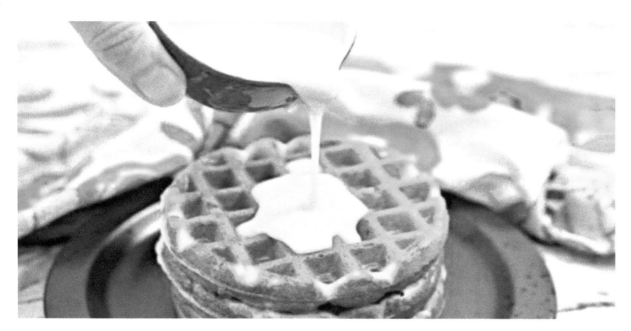

15 mins

Servings 3

Ingredients:

For the chaffles:

- ½ cup Mozzarella cheese shredded
- 1 ounce Cream Cheese
- 2 tablespoon Unflavored whey protein isolate
- 2 tablespoon Swerve confectioners sugar substitute
- ½ teaspoon Baking powder
- ½ teaspoon Vanilla extract
- 1 Egg

For the glaze topping:

- 2 tablespoon Heavy whipping cream
- 3-4 tablespoon Swerve confectioners sugar substitute
- ½ teaspoon Vanilla extract

Preparation:

1. Preheat your waffle maker for mini waffles.

2. Combine the mozzarella and cream cheese in a microwave-safe dish. Heat for 30 seconds at a time before the cheeses are fully melted and mixed.

3. Toss the cheese mixture with the whey protein, 2 tbsp Swerve confectioners sweetener, and baking powder, and knead with your hands until well combined.

4. In a mixing bowl, whisk together the dough, egg, and vanilla extract until a smooth batter forms.

5. Place a third of the batter in the mini waffle maker and cook for 3-5 minutes, or until desired doneness is achieved.

6. Repeat the procedure 5 and 6 with the remaining 2/3 of the batter to make 3 chaffles.

7. To make the glaze topping, whisk together all of the ingredients and pour over the chaffles just before serving.

WAFFLE WITH VANILLA AND COCONUT AND STRAWBERRY, BANANA AND MAPLE YOGURT

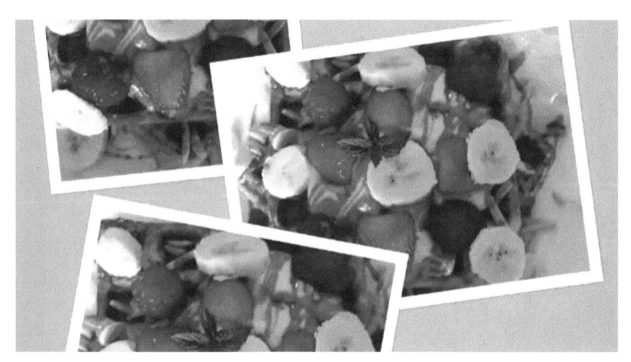

Time required: 3-5 min

Portions provided: 4-6

Ingredients:

- cups brown rice flour
- 1/2 cup of coconut flour
- 1/4 teaspoon murray river sea salt
- 2 teaspoons baking powder
- cups unsweetened almond milk
- 1 scoop of protein powder of your choice (optional)
- 2 eggs
- 4 tablespoons coconut oil
- 1 tablespoon maple syrup
- 50 g each of blueberries, raspberries, and strawberries
- Olive/coconut oil spray

Preparation:

1. A waffle iron with a high heat environment.

2. Combine all of the dry ingredients in a mixing bowl.

3. Combine the milk, coconut oil, and eggs in a mixing bowl. Combine the dry and wet ingredients in a mixing bowl. To achieve a batter consistency, add a little more milk.

4. Spray the waffle iron lightly with the spray. Pour batter into waffle iron and cook for 3 to 5 minutes, or until finished.

5. Serve with fruit, maple syrup made from bananas, and a dollop of vanilla coconut yogurt.

6. Recognize: you can freeze the leftover wafers between parchment paper in the freezer.

7. Note: if you're using protein powder, add another 1/4 cup almond milk to keep the mixture from being too thick.

KETO CHAFFLE YOGURT

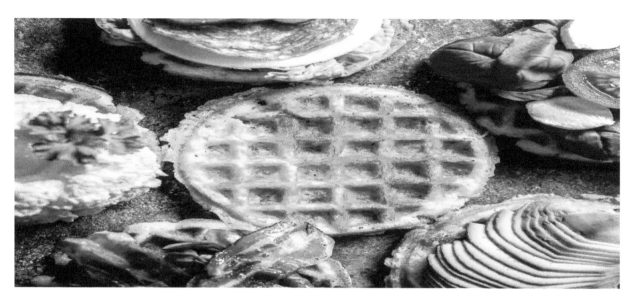

Time required: 17 min

Portions provided: 4

Ingredients:

- 1/2 cup (50 g) mozzarella cheese
- 1 egg
- 2 tablespoons (17 g) ground almonds
- 1/2 teaspoon (1.5 g) psyllium husk
- 1 g (1/4 teaspoon) baking powder
- 1 tablespoon (20 g) yogurt

Preparation:

1. Heat your waffle iron and prepare all of the ingredients.

2. To soften the chaffles, finely slice the mozzarella.

3. To begin, beat the eggs with a fork in a cup.

4. Mix in the remaining ingredients, except the mozzarella. Mix in the sliced mozzarella after the batter has been thoroughly cooked.

5. Allow for a few minutes for the physilium to function on its own.

6. Spray the waffle iron gently with oil if it doesn't have a non-stick coating.

7. We suggest grated cheese on the bottom of the waffle iron for perfectly crispy chaffles.

8. In the center of the cheese, place a big tablespoon of pasta. If you add too many, the chaffle will scatter across the vehicle.

9. Grading

10. It's much easier to use finely grated cheese.

11. Cook for 3-4 minutes, or until they stop smoking.

12. Using freshly grated cheese instead, since it includes additives and flour to prevent the bits from sticking together.

13. For a crispier note, sprinkle grated cheese on top and bottom of the plate.

14. Just use egg whites to replace the whole egg if you think it's too much egg for you.

15. Cook it for a longer time if you like it crispier.

16. While the chaffle maker is smoking, do not attempt to open it. It's possible the chaffle would fall apart.

Nutrition Facts: *Per Serving:* Calories 93; Carbohydrates 2g; Total Fat 5g

REAL FOOD CHOCOLATE WAFFLES

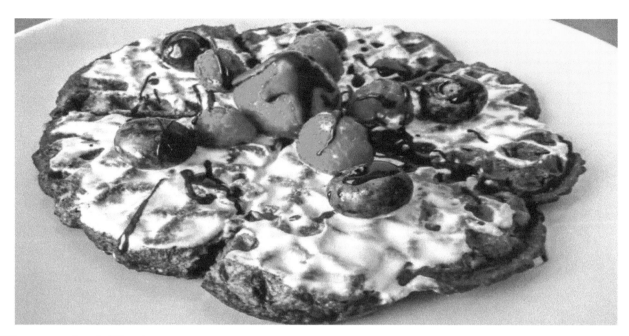

Time required: 20 min

Portions provided: 4

Ingredients:

- 220 gr rolled oats or oatmeal
- 3 bananas
- 4 eggs
- 6 natural pitted dates
- 50 ml oatmeal drink
- 40 gr pure cocoa powder type valor
- 1 tablespoon ground cinnamon
- 2 pinches baking soda
- 1 dash lemon
- 1/2 envelope (8 gr) chemical yeast (if you don't have baking soda)

Toppings (optional and to taste):

- 2-3 teaspoons whipped cheese 0% fat
- 1 ripe strawberry
- 5 raspberries
- 5 blueberries
- 1 large ounce chocolate 85% and up

Preparation:

1. In a blender, efficient processor, or robot, combine the dough ingredients and blend for 1 minute on speed 5-6, or until all is chopped and well combined. Put the medium on the yeast or the bicarbonate and the lemon splash to lighten it up, but not both at the same time.

2. When the waffle iron is hot, add 3 heaping tablespoons of the mixture to the center and bake. Two heaping tablespoons fit in each hole if there are two holes.

3. Close it and wait for the green light to turn on after the key. I gave myself a 3 out of 5 on this stage.

4. Although it is delicious as is, you can customize it with your favorite toppings and enjoy!!

STRAWBERRIES & CREAM KETO CHAFFLES

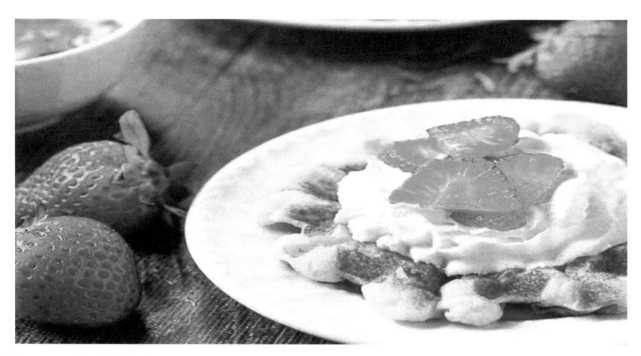

Time required: 35 min

Portions provided: 2

Ingredients:

- 3 oz cream cheese
- 2 cups mozzarella cheese, shredded
- 2 eggs, beaten
- 1/2 cup almond flour
- 3 tablespoons Swerve confectioners sweetener
- 2 teaspoons baking powder
- 8 strawberries
- 1 cup whipped cream (canister - 2 tablespoons per waffle)
- 1 tablespoon Swerve confectioners sweetener

Preparation:

1. Microwave the cream cheese and mozzarella for 1 minute in a microwave-safe dish.

2. Mix thoroughly, then proceed to the next stage if any of the cheese has melted. Otherwise, cook for another 30 seconds and then thoroughly mix. In a separate cup, whisk together the eggs, then add the almond flour, baking powder, and 3 tablespoons Swerve sweetener.

3. Mix well the cream cheese mixture with the almond flour mixture, then fold in two sliced strawberries. Refrigerate for 20 minutes before serving.

4. Meanwhile, dice the remaining strawberries and add 1 tablespoon of Swerve to the mixture. Set aside or refrigerate after thoroughly mixing.

5. Remove the batter from the refrigerator after 20 minutes. Warm up your waffle iron, and if it needs to be greased, do so.

6. 1/4 cup of the mixture should be placed in the center of a hot waffle iron. Make the waffles as small as possible to make them easier to remove from the waffle maker.

7. Move to a plate and set aside to cool before topping with whipped cream and strawberries.

8. I got 8 tiny waffles out of this recipe.

Nutrition Facts: *For 1 waffle with strawberries and cream:* Calories 189; Carbohydrates 5.2g; Fat 14,3g; Fiber 1g; Protein 10g

BLUEBERRY CHAFFLES

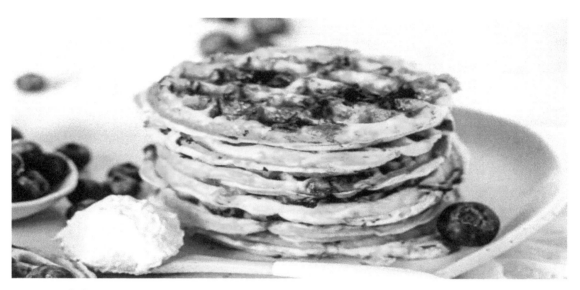

Time required: 30 min

Portions provided: 4

Ingredients:

- 4 eggs
- 1 cup (4 oz.) shredded mozzarella cheese
- 1 tbsp coconut flour
- 1 tsp vanilla extract
- 3 oz. (9 1/3 tbsp) fresh blueberries
- Serving
- ½ cup heavy whipping cream
- 6 oz. (1 1/5 cups) fresh blueberries

Preparation:

1. Warm up your waffle iron.

2. In a mixing bowl, combine all of your ingredients and beat to combine.

3. Allow for a 5-minute rest period to allow the coconut flour to absorb some moisture.

4. Spread the mixture uniformly over the bottom plate of your waffle iron, spacing it out slightly to get an even result. Close the waffle iron and cook for 6 minutes, depending on the waffle maker you have.

5. When you think they're done, gently raise the lid.

6. Serve with new blueberries and strong whipping cream.

7. hints

8. When the chaffles are finished, they can easily release from the waffle iron. The blueberries, on the other hand, ooze a bit of sweet juice, which causes the chaffle to stick. You will need to use a spatula to gently lift them off the waffle iron.

9. These chaffles are best served immediately, but they can also be frozen and reheated.

10. A sweet, sugar-free, warm berry syrup can be made by heating fresh blueberries in the microwave for 30 or 40 seconds to a minute.

LOW D FRENCH TOAST WAFFLES

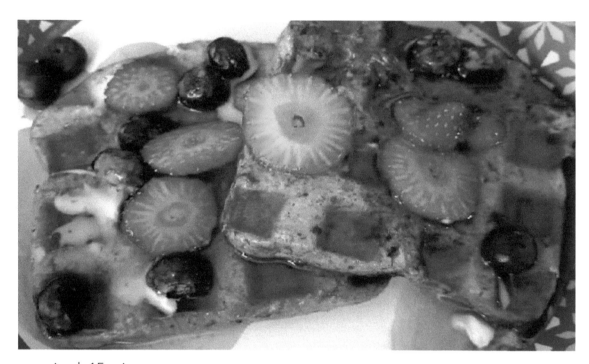

Time required: 15 min

Portions provided: 1

Ingredients:

- 2 discs zero
- Carbohydrate bread
- 1 large egg
- 1/8 cup unsweetened almond milk
- 1/4 teaspoon cinnamon
- 2 strawberries, sliced
- 8-10 blueberries

Preparation:

1. In a mixing bowl, whisk together the egg, almond milk, and cinnamon.
2. Bread should be dipped into the egg mixture.
3. Use a waffle iron to make the waffles.
4. Garnish with berries and maple syrup that hasn't been sweetened.

HEALTHY BERRY WAFFLES

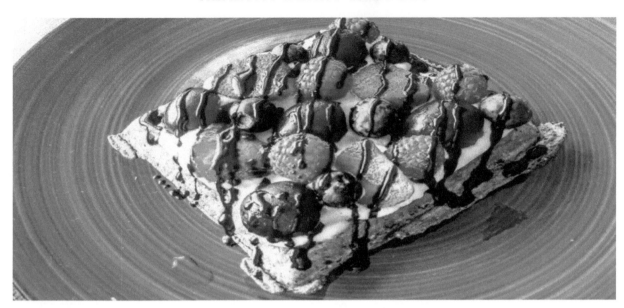

Time required: 20 min

Portions provided: 8

Ingredients:

- 220 gr rolled oats or whole oatmeal
- 4 eggs (I use free range)
- 2 bananas
- 6 natural pitted dates (optional)
- 2 pinches baking soda
- 1 good squirt of lemon juice
- 1 tablespoon ground cinnamon
- 1 tablespoon cranberry powder (optional)

Topping:
- 1 level tablespoon fresh cheese whipped 0% fat (optional)
- 1 strawberry
- 3 cherries
- 5 raspberries
- 6 blueberries
- 1 ounce chocolate 85%-90%

Preparation:

1. Place the ingredients in the robot's or blender's glass.

2. Blend until you have smooth, lump-free dough. At speed 5-6, it takes about 1 minute on the robot. When the light comes on in the waffle iron, pour two tablespoons of batter into the middle of each hole.

3. The waffles are ready when the green light on the waffle maker clicks on and the click sounds.

4. With a spatula, remove them from the pan and top with the red fruits and a tablespoon of whipped fresh cheese (if using).

5. For each waffle, microwave one ounce of chocolate with at least 85 percent cocoa. With a teaspoon, spread it over the end. And have a great time!!

Thank you for reading this book.
If you enjoyed it, please visit the site where you purchased it and write a brief review. Your feedback is important to me and will help other readers decide whether to read the book too.

Thank you!
Susan Lombardi

CPSIA information can be obtained
at www.ICGtesting.com
Printed in the USA
LVHW071256281221
707346LV00025B/468

9 781802 172591